if memory serves me wrong

A memoir of theatre,
love and loss to
early-onset Alzheimer's

RONAN SMITH

with SUE LEONARD
Foreword by Professor Ian Robertson

NEW ISLAND

IF MEMORY SERVES ME WRONG
First published in 2021 by
New Island Books
Glenshesk House
10 Richview Office Park
Clonskeagh
Dublin D14 V8C4
Republic of Ireland
www.newisland.ie

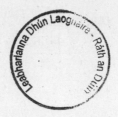

Print ISBN: 978-1-84840-807-4
eBook ISBN: 978-1-84840-808-1

Typeset by JVR Creative India
Cover design by Fiachra McCarthy, fiachramccarthy.com
Edited by Susan McKeever, susanmckeever.biz
Indexed by Jane Rogers
Printed by L&C Printing Group, Poland

New Island Books is a member of Publishing Ireland.

10 9 8 7 6 5 4 3 2 1

if memory serves me wrong

To Miriam, Hannah and Loughlin, with deepest love.

DNA neither cares nor knows.
DNA just is. And we dance to its music.
—*Richard Dawkins*

Contents

Foreword

Ian Robertson, Emeritus Professor of Psychology in Trinity College Dublin and Co-Director of the Global Brain Health Institute

When Ronan Smith spoke to Gay Byrne on *The Late Late Show* in 1989 about his father Brendan's Alzheimer's disease, it was the first time that the closet doors of stigma and denial surrounding this disease had been thrown open so widely. Ronan's pioneering leadership in the early years of the Alzheimer Society of Ireland (ASI), and his crucial work as an advocate for families afflicted with Alzheimer's disease, are part of his proud and lasting legacy. When Ronan himself was diagnosed with the same, rare early-onset version of the disease as his father, that legacy grew as he used his intelligence, courage and commitment to resume his advocacy work, including as chair of the ASI's Dementia Working Group.

At a time now where scarcely an Irish family is untouched by the illness, Ronan's story of caring for his father, and then facing the same disease himself, could not be more timely. This book is unique and important because it tells the story of dementia from both sides, inside and out. But this is much more than a memoir about a very, very tough disease – it is also a tale of bravery, loyalty and love.

How, you might ask, could a book about Alzheimer's disease be as beautiful, interesting and funny as it is hauntingly sad?

Maybe only if it is written by two highly intelligent, insightful and empathic people trying their best to live with the hand that nature has dealt them. For this is as much a poignant love story as it is a tale of fate wielding its brutal club.

Ronan has early-onset Alzheimer's disease, and his wife Miriam's hilarious account of the unravelling of a blameless lie would on its own make this book worth reading for even the least dementia-interested reader. Instructing her producer and actor husband Ronan to tell a caller that she was in bed asleep, she ends up in a string of hilarious conundrums – theatrical farce as funny as the best that Dublin's Gaiety Theatre ever presented.

The Olympia Theatre sits squarely centre-stage in this story. It is here that the young Ronan first has the awful realisation that his larger-than-life father – director of the Olympia and of the Dublin Theatre Festival – is unravelling chaotically in front of his eyes, brought low by Alzheimer's disease. Hopelessly in denial, he is threatening to bring down the jewels of Dublin's theatrical firmament with him. And it is in another Dublin theatre, The Gaiety, that Ronan finally retires from a career in Irish and international theatre that spanned the Abbey to Broadway, and *The Pirate Queen* to *Riverdance*.

With this rich and vibrant backdrop, you would want to read this story even if you had never heard of Alzheimer's disease. But this is much, much more than the memoir of two remarkable thespians. The book lures you in because it is so well-written, interesting and funny. Then, softly but expertly, it punches you in the guts. It brings you face to face with what you shy away from because you dread it so much – your own dissolution.

This is a tale that is mythical and eternal, of great love tested by brute, biological reality. A rogue gene inherited from his father seeds Ronan's brain with shards of toxic protein that gnaw at his day-to-day memory and steal his beautiful words.

Miriam's voice interweaves with Ronan's, a pure love haunted by illness and by the slow fading of her husband's brilliance, her words becoming more pain-wracked yet ever more loving.

It is a sad truth that most of us will become characters in some version of a story like this, but there is hope on the horizon for the new treatments that will arrive for such diseases. Artificial intelligence, for example, has recently unfurled the mystery of how proteins fold. We can have hope – or even confidence – that eventually the rogue proteins in our brains can be packed away and forgotten.

But while we impatiently await these scientific advances, we need to better understand this disease and its impacts on families, to better support them and give them the quality of life they deserve. This unique book makes one giant step towards this goal, and we owe Ronan and Miriam a real debt of gratitude for their courage in writing it.

Prologue

It was my sixtieth birthday, and my wife had organised a party. I'd been expecting an intimate affair, but Miriam surprised me with a stay in the beautiful Tinakilly House Hotel in Co. Wicklow, where we were joined by ninety guests from all the different spheres of my life. Along with my children, Hannah and Loughlin, my brother Julian and his family, friends from college and some neighbours, there were many from the world of theatre – including a cluster who had acted with Miriam on RTÉ's *Glenroe*. Some had travelled a great distance. I felt like the surprised guest on *This Is Your Life*.

Miriam had thought of everything. Wonderful tapas arrived throughout the evening, the wine flowed and the band played on. Two close friends spoke; Martin Drury gave me a eulogy – there is no other word for it – and Philip Lee gave a speech that doubled as a comic routine. When Hannah and Loughlin stood up and sang a song to me in harmony, I thought that the evening couldn't get any better. But then it did.

The room darkened, and lights flashed as the sound of thunder slowly filled the room. As the sound rose, vibrating around us, we looked at each other in alarm, but then the double doors at the top of the room burst open, and in came a troupe of dancers, their feet taking up the drumming, thundery sound as they reached the recently constructed stage. It was the *Riverdance* Flying Squad, I realised. I stared at them open-mouthed, then I looked at Miriam, who was smiling broadly.

'How?' I asked. 'When?'

Then John McColgan and Moya Doherty, the founders of *Riverdance*, whom I had worked with so closely over the years, tapped me on the shoulder and said, 'Happy birthday, Ronan. This is our gift to you.'

When the male dancers had completed the 'Thunderstorm' routine they were joined by the females as they broke into 'Riverdance', the number that had taken the world by storm as the interval act of the Eurovision Song Contest in 1994. I must have watched that memorable performance hundreds of times when I was overseeing *Riverdance*'s many overseas productions, but such was the impact of those thirty dancers in this small room, it was as if I was seeing and hearing it for the first time. And judging from the emotion I witnessed on the faces of those around me, it was clear that my friends were finding the performance just as electrifying as I was.

'You're amazing,' I said to Miriam as the performance drew to a close. 'How did you plan that?'

'With a lot of help,' she said, indicating Julian Erskine, who had been lighting the performance from across the room. 'He and I have been working on this for months. I couldn't have done it without him.'

I smiled, delighted at this show of real friendship. Then Miriam took to the stage. I was amazed. Although she's an excellent actor, Miriam is shy, and speaking in public is an ordeal for her. But she was wonderful. Starting out by thanking everyone, especially Julian Erskine, she then told a story.

When our children were seven and five, they'd come into our bed at weekends. And one morning Hannah, being a daddy's girl, started telling Ronan how much she loved him. She went on and on and Ronan, who was loving this, asked her why. 'Because you're so tidy,' she said. 'And so neat. And so clever. And you work so hard.'

I tried not to ask the question, but I was feeling jealous and I couldn't stop myself. I said, 'Hannah, do you love Mummy?'

'Um … um, yeah, I suppose.'

She didn't sound so sure, so again, knowing I shouldn't, I asked her why she loved me.

'I don't know.' She furrowed her brow. Then, her face brightening, she said, 'Yes I do! I know why. You make really good decisions.'

'Do I?'

'Yeah. You decided to marry Daddy.'

The room erupted into laughter. And then music came on, playing gently. It was Barry White singing 'You're the First, the Last, My Everything', and over the music Miriam, turning, looked at me and said, 'And Ronan, Hannah was right. I *do* make good decisions, and marrying you was the best one I ever made.'

I went up to her and we embraced. Then Hannah and Loughlin joined us in a group hug, and Miriam and I danced. And I thought I would burst with happiness.

As we sat relaxing by the fire in the small hours, I thought what a perfect night it had been; one I would look back on and remember for the rest of my life. And then, with a shock, I realised that I *wouldn't* remember it. Not with my diagnosis. Not with my early-onset Alzheimer's.

One

A Day in Ronan's Life: November 2019

I wake early and have no idea what day it is. That's not unusual – in fact it's the case every morning now. Since I was diagnosed with early-onset Alzheimer's disease in 2014, my short-term memory has been letting me down, and it's getting worse. It's the first area the illness attacks. I can remember things from my childhood, but cannot begin to recall what I did an hour and a half ago.

Leaving my wife Miriam to sleep a little longer, I get up and go out to the kitchen. I've missed the sunrise, but the morning light shimmers through the trees, lighting up Blessington Lake, which provides a pleasing contrast to the shadowy Wicklow hills on the horizon.

My first task of the day is to feed the hens, a job I love. There are currently six of them, of different varieties, including Rhode Island Red. Wild excitement breaks out, with lots of squawking, when I go into their quarter-acre pen and throw the corn. I collect the eggs, which are still warm to the touch. We used to have pigs – we had three and reared them for the freezer – but they were a lot of work, and around the time of my diagnosis we decided that we wouldn't have them again.

Returning to the house, I make my breakfast. It's always something hot. Sometimes I have beans on toast, or an egg, but today I fry up some bread, and put some tomatoes on the pan. I eat that with some goat's cheese. It's delicious.

I turn on the radio and listen to *Morning Ireland*. There's been yet another murder in Dublin. The Gardaí suspect that it was carried out by a rival drug gang. When, at nine o'clock, Ryan Tubridy comes on, I listen to the introduction where he does a roundup of the day, then I switch off.

I make the coffee as Miriam walks through the door, yawning. This once-simple task is becoming confusing to me. It's because my sequencing is breaking down.

'It's because there are so many stages involved in making coffee,' explains Miriam. 'You have to find the bag of coffee, then get out the pot. Then there's the boiling water to think about, and the pot has to be opened and closed again.'

The process sounds so simple when she says it, but she's right. I catch myself staring at the coffee grounds, wondering if I should spoon them straight into the cup. It can take time to figure out the lid of the pot. Today I manage it all, then go to the fridge for the milk. There's another decision to be made. Should we have the protein milk, the soya or the almond?

While we drink our coffee, and Miriam tucks into her breakfast, we go through our diaries. There's an entry in mine where I've written, '11.30 a.m: Martin Drury to visit'. He's a close and loyal friend. Yesterday I had a meeting with the Dementia Working Group, as part of the Alzheimer Society of Ireland (ASI), in Brooks Hotel in Dublin. I'm chair of the group, which is made up of people who have the illness.

It's important to me to contribute to the advocacy message, as it's made a significant change in reducing stigma around the disease. When my father, the theatre impresario Brendan Smith, contracted Alzheimer's there was shame around the issue and, perhaps as a consequence, he hid his illness and never acknowledged that there was anything wrong with him. It was a mistake, and one I am anxious not to repeat.

Many of the people attending the meeting were accompanied by carers, but I travelled in alone by bus. Miriam dropped me at the stop at Blessington. I made my way in without difficulty, I got off at the right bus stop and headed for Brooks Hotel but, for a moment, I hadn't a clue where I was. It was very strange. I couldn't orientate myself. The streetscape confused me, and standing there I thought, 'Shit! I can't find the hotel, but I know it's somewhere around here.'

I stood there, gave myself time and worked out that it wasn't down the road to my right, nor the one to my left, and by going straight I found my bearings again. The meeting was surprisingly good-humoured. Occasionally a new member will be full of anger, but yesterday was uplifting. There was much laughter as people vied to tell the best Alzheimer's bad joke. When I arrived home, Miriam asked me what I'd done with my coat, and I realised I'd left it back there in the hotel.

After breakfast I call the dogs and go out for my morning walk. Bella, our young Cockapoo, is ready at once. She has been bouncing around my heels for some time, carrying a sock. But Pepsi, an old fella like me, who is deaf and I swear has dementia, is lying on a bed somewhere and has to be fetched.

Pepsi is a rescue dog who came to us when our son Loughlin was small, and *he's* now at NCAD – the National College of Art and Design in Dublin. I start out, but have to return because I've forgotten Bella's lead; then we make our way down, through a local farm to the beach at the lake's edge. I love it there, gazing out as the dogs run around, playing. Bella jumps all over Pepsi and soon tires him out. I can spend an hour at a time there, thinking, taking in the scenery.

When I get home I make some green tea and go through to my office. I take my first tranche of pills. I'm on a cocktail of Alzheimer's drugs that needs to be taken twice a day, and I'm currently also taking pills for my unsettled tummy. In an effort to counteract that, and to ease my nausea, I'm experimenting by eating little and often.

I'm very keen to stay active mentally as well as physically, and my writing project has become an obsession. Today I'm having trouble spelling words. That's new – I normally don't have to think about it – and I try to remember, determined not to 'give in' and look at a dictionary. I spend a minute or so toying with the word. It's no good. I look the word up. That worries me, but I've learned from experience that it doesn't necessarily mean I've lost that facility forever. Tomorrow I might have no difficulty with my spelling at all.

At eleven o'clock I make myself a snack. I have tomatoes and goat's cheese in a bun. Miriam comes in and says, 'You had the same for breakfast,' and I tell her it's healthy, so what's the problem?

'But Ronan, cheese is not great for your cholesterol. Remember, the doctor said to watch it?'

I don't understand. 'But I'm eating little and often.'

'I know. But if you have more fat now, it will affect your high blood pressure.'

I get pissed off then. I can't help it. But I give in, put the goat's cheese aside, and eat the banana sandwich Miriam makes for me instead. Loughlin comes into the kitchen at that point. It's his college holidays and he's come home to help Miriam in the garden. He asks what we're talking about.

'Food,' I say.

'The other week your father made himself toast with Nutella on it,' says Miriam. 'Do you remember, Ronan?'

I nod. 'Nothing wrong with Nutella.'

'No. Except it was something you never used to eat. Oh, and you put tomato chutney on top of the Nutella.'

'Dad – you didn't! That's gross!'

'But it tasted good,' I say.

Miriam laughs. 'And then, last week, you had toast and chorizo and sardines – with raspberry jam on top.'

I shrug and say, 'That's one of the pluses of having Alzheimer's, and there aren't too many of those.' I turn to my son. 'I'm trying to be good. And my carer is pretty problematic, actually.'

We laugh. Well, you have to. It's either that sometimes, or cry.

'I think I'll go back to my office until lunchtime,' I say, turning to leave the kitchen.

'But it's 11.30,' says Miriam.

I narrow my eyes questioningly.

'Martin Drury is coming.'

'Is he? Why didn't you tell me?'

'I did.'

It's good to see Martin, who is full of theatre chat – telling me what our mutual friends are up to. We became close in college and have been friends and colleagues since, and I miss the world of the theatre. I can't even remember when I last saw a play. I seem to have lost my appetite for it, as I have lost my appetite for so many things.

Martin goes before lunch and afterwards I take the dogs for a second walk, going up the road this time, to catch a better view. When I return, I decide to do a little gardening. Miriam is the expert – I'm just the commis gardener and do what I am told. I have to be careful now with machinery. I can use the sit-on mower because the engine turns off automatically when you climb off it, but I was using the push mower recently and misjudged things, putting my hand in to clear the blades when the machine was still running. I cut my finger badly and it took a good few visits to plastics in St James's to sort it out. The nail has grown since, but I have to be honest with myself and accept my limitations. I now avoid anything mechanised. Today I weed the driveway by hand. I know I could spray weedkiller over it, but I find picking out the grass and weeds strangely meditative. I police the gravel, making it my business to keep it in check.

I spend a lot of the day looking for things that I've lost. I know this happens to everyone to some extent, but it's magnified for me and can be extremely frustrating. I normally lose my glasses or my phone, but today it's my wallet. Miriam and I have searched everywhere, and we can't find it. Should we cancel my credit cards?

Simple tasks take me longer. Miriam says that I spend much too long in the kitchen, wiping the surfaces repeatedly, or running the tap over a spoon for ages before I put it in the dishwasher. I think I'm simply being thorough. When we're going somewhere in the car, I get wired up gathering all my things together, making sure I have everything on Miriam's checklist – the days are over when I can just leave the house without a thought.

When I first got the diagnosis, Miriam and I discussed how I could best fight the illness. Miriam explored ways to help slow the disease down and conducted research into diet and exercise for Alzheimer's.

On her regime, I take as much exercise as possible. Miriam takes me to a local swimming pool twice or three times a week. I go hillwalking with a group sometimes, staying out for four or five hours. I cycle too, and Miriam is enrolling me on a badminton course for the autumn. It will be good for my coordination.

We decided to take on a ketogenic diet. It's extremely healthy – we consume very little red meat. Tonight we eat fish, with organic spinach, courgettes and mangetout, picked fresh from the garden. These days I eat it in front of the six o'clock news. I don't read a newspaper. I never really did, but I make sure to see the news every evening.

I've become a little bit obsessed with the whole Brexit thing. I find it just so alarming and extraordinary, and I'm gobsmacked at the behaviour of people. I still think there's a possibility that Britain won't leave the European Union. The fact that Boris Johnson only has one vote, it would be a very serious thing to take Britain out under those circumstances.

It's a fine August evening, and I take a glass of red wine and walk up the garden to Miriam's borders. It's peaceful there, sitting on a bench. It's like looking at a stage or perhaps at an audience, as the lawn falls away, and the view past the house to the water beyond is so beautiful. I sit, sip my wine and watch the clouds form shapes in that enormous expanse of sky, and I let my mind drift.

When I come in I watch some TV, but it's hard these days to keep up. I can, mostly, follow a given episode of a drama, but I don't remember what happened before this episode. It's a very frustrating problem. And when there are sophisticated ruses to throw the audience off like, for example, in *Peaky Blinders*, I go, 'Fuck!' I just watch it and remember, vaguely, who all the characters are. Documentaries are easier to follow.

I read in bed every night before I settle to sleep. I find reading books easier than watching films and television, because I can always go back and check who people are and what has happened. I've recently read and enjoyed Colum McCann's *Let the Great World Spin* and *A Suitable Boy* by Vikram Seth. I'm now reading a book by a woman who cared for her father, who had dementia.

I was cautious at first, but reading it has been fine, and very real and telling. It shows how awkward and awful the journey can be, but I already know that from dealing with my father. Still, I'm glad I started it, and am happy to continue to read it. I'm a little critical of some of the things she says, occasionally going, 'No, I don't think that's right.'

I subscribe to *National Geographic*, and I love that. There's such a range of subjects, and I'm interested in all the countries and issues the magazine covers. I appreciate the wonderful journalism produced by that organisation, and I like the fact that you can read a whole article with a beginning, a middle and an end. I love the experience of reading it and, though I can't retain all I've read and know I won't remember the half of it, I enjoy it at the time.

We've had to make a lot of adjustments as a couple since my diagnosis. Miriam is still my lover as well as my carer. We have to be careful to keep that balance and not drift apart in some effort to protect each other. I know she often feels upset. I hear her crying at night and do my best to comfort her.

I try not to despair. Ninety per cent of the time I manage to be reconciled to what has happened. None of this is my fault. I haven't done anything wrong. The condition has arrived, and it is beginning to have an increasing impact. I have a certain understanding of the illness, but I'm not burdening myself with the facts. I sleep well, and if I wake in the night I have no trouble dropping off to sleep again.

Two

Beginnings

I can't claim that I was close to my father; I barely knew him when I was a child. I was born in Dublin on 29 November 1957, two years after the arrival of my brother Julian. By this time both my parents, Brendan Smith and Beryl Fagan, were entirely committed to, and even obsessed with, professional theatre.

There were to be no other siblings – unless of course you count the most important one – namely the Dublin Theatre Festival, which was founded by my father in the same year that I was born. I have come to see it, superstitiously, as some sort of lifelong twin. Its fortunes, a little like mine, drifted up and down from year to year.

It was also a demanding child, claiming so much of my father's time and energy that he was rarely in the house. He spent his days in the office and his evenings taking in a show. And when he was at home, he didn't engage with Julian or me. He was distant and remote. I don't think he knew quite what to do with us.

My mother was more of a presence in our lives. She was the one giving us affection and taking an interest in all that we did, but she shared with my father the glamour and excitement of the theatrical life. She was a professional actress with a particular love of musicals, and also a radio presenter.

As my childhood progressed and my father's achievements, along with his status, began to grow, she was out with him on social engagements more and more. She also lent a hand in the Brendan Smith Theatre Academy, which my father had founded back in 1941.

Thanks partly to his childhood circumstances, theatre was in my father's blood. In the early 1930s his mother, Greta Smith, started working at the Gate Theatre in Dublin, playing the cello during the half hour before the curtain rose to entertain the audience as it drifted in. Because she was a widow she needed the income from this, and a second job, in order to support herself and her two children.

This was the time of Hilton Edwards and Micheál Mac Liammóir, the eccentric but highly celebrated stars of Irish theatre who were based at the Gate Theatre. Audiences loved them, relishing the plays which were considered more exciting than the more conservative fare dished up by the Abbey Theatre. The two theatres were acknowledged rivals. A wit of the time referred to the two as Sodom and Begorrah.

My father attended Belvedere, a school geographically convenient to the Gate Theatre. The Jesuits had provided him with a charity scholarship, and he'd walk from the school to the Gate to be babysat by the house staff until his mother arrived from her other job. Hilton Edwards let my father sit beside him to watch rehearsals and auditions, and in that way he learned the basics of theatre from a highly skilled director in an entirely casual and unstructured way.

The Brendan Smith Theatre Academy had a senior and a junior section and, naturally enough, Julian and I were both enrolled into the children's classes. I loved it – and got a tremendous buzz from performing – but Julian suffered there horribly. There's a photograph of us taken at one of the Academy shows when I was about seven or eight years old, showing me dressed as an elf, and Julian as an Indian with a blacked-out face. I'm beaming from ear to ear, but poor Julian looks miserable. It was a terrible mistake, in my view, to foist the classes on him. Yet they persevered in making him attend. I can remember him saying to me later in life, 'You came into the world as an actor.' It was very clear that he did not.

But those were different times, and my father was keen that we should be given an opportunity to develop in something that was his passion. And back then, acting schools for kids were generally attended by a mix of children: those who loved performing, and those who were being made to go by ambitious parents. We went there every Saturday afternoon for classes, and we performed scenes from plays with regularity.

I also took part in some television and radio advertisements at a young age. In one advertisement I had to say, 'Sometimes my mum flies off the handle.' That was my line and, although I said it a tedious number of times, I didn't know what it meant!

My mother employed a series of live-in housekeepers that came and went over the years of my childhood. She came from a comfortable middle-class background so the concept of paid help felt appropriate to her, but my friends found the setup strange. They'd come to play and say, 'Who is this? It's not your mum.' And I'd have to explain.

We lived in Marlborough Road, Donnybrook but, unlike the grand three-storey Georgian houses the road is known for, our house was modern and, being relatively small, wasn't grand enough to make such an *Upstairs, Downstairs* arrangement practical. The housekeeper's room was small and, in retrospect, I realise the incumbents lived an isolated life. Most of them came from the country and were from a sad platoon of those females who have to leave the farm because there is no longer a place for them. I never felt that their hearts were in the job; they were probably unhappy and disappointed people.

The best of them, Miss Ritchie, was there for the early years of my life. She was very formal and proper. When she tucked us into bed she pulled the sheets and blankets as tight as she could, and left, saying, 'Do not get out of this bed!' But she was conscientious, and my parents knew they could rely on her. When she handed in her notice, my mother was distraught.

'But you can't go! What will I do without you?' she said, begging her to change her mind. 'Are you not happy here?'

'They need me at home,' she said. 'I have to care for my mother.' There really was no arguing with that.

Miss F, who arrived some years later, delighted in teasing Julian and his friends about girls. It was totally inappropriate to do this to an adolescent, and it appalled and embarrassed him. But she wasn't as bad as the one who arrived in the household when I was nine years old.

Soon after she arrived, Julian and I had been out visiting a friend. When we were delivered home and the housekeeper opened the door to us, her speech sounded strange. 'Ah, there you are,' she said, whooshing us inside. 'Off you go now, off you go!'

She said goodbye as she waved off our friend and his mother, and we watched as they walked to their car and drove off. But the housekeeper, keeping the door open, was still talking. Julian and I looked at each other in alarm.

'Thank you very much,' she was saying, addressing thin air. 'Thank you very, very, very, very much. Thank you.'

What was going on? Eventually she shut the door and came in, but she wobbled a bit and was decidedly unsteady on her feet. Falling backwards, she slumped into an armchair and was soon snoring, her mouth open.

Realising that she was incapable from drink, we put ourselves to bed that night. I'm not sure how my parents got to hear of this, but soon, that housekeeper was history.

It was a relief when there was no longer a need for a live-in housekeeper, and instead we had someone who would come in and work between certain set hours.

Julian and I were good pals. We shared a room in harmony, except when he wanted to keep reading and I did not. On Saturdays we used to toss a coin to see who went for their bath first, because that's when *Batman* was on. We hated missing it, but with the washing schedule, neither of us could watch the full programme. We'd each get half of it, and we had to brief each other on the plot as we passed each other in the corridor. He would say, 'Batman and Robin are fighting the Riddler,' and meanwhile the housekeeper would be shouting, 'Will you come up the stairs!'

As small boys Julian and I were in the same local gang, along with three others. Julian was the brains who would find ways to frustrate the enemy – the strategist of the operation. When we weren't taking on our rivals on the street, we'd get up to mischief in the gardens. Each of the houses had a rear entrance with a single door. We could climb over the wall, and we'd do that often, to rob apples. Sometimes we took my mother's stockings and stuffed them with apples or stones. We'd swing them then let go and see who could throw theirs the furthest. One time, mine flew over the neighbour's wall. I was delighted, until the lady came and roared at me over the fence.

'You could have killed my baby.' Red-faced with anger, she shook her fists at me, and I was terrified for my life. It turned out the infant was sleeping in his pram, and my stocking of stones had missed him by inches. I didn't try that one again.

When we left for school in the mornings my parents were still in bed. They'd have breakfast served to them upstairs – in their separate rooms. My mother, I always understood, was highly strung; a euphemism, I now know, for being anxious or depressed. Sometimes when we got home from school, we'd find her in bed. Bemused, I'd ask her why she was there and she'd say, 'I'm not well.'

'Will you be better tomorrow?'

She'd answer with something non-committal. Then came the time that she disappeared into a nursing home. When, concerned, we asked Dad why, the answer was, 'Your mother needs to have a rest. She will be home again soon.'

We visited. She was pleased to see us, but her speech sounded slurred. She was on heavy medication, and it was clearly a struggle for her to engage with us. She made an effort though, listening carefully to our childhood chatter and asking questions as we told her how the cat was, and what we were up to at school.

As we became older, we began to see a pattern to her illness. She'd get the blues, take to the bed, maybe go to a nursing home, then she'd pick herself up again. It was just another thing that went on in our house, and as a child you just accepted it.

We took the glamour of thespian life in our stride too. Every Christmas we visited other theatre people. Hugh Leonard – whose real name was Jack Keyes Byrne – was a great friend, although my parents' relationship with him and his wife Paula was an ambiguous one. Jack's cantankerousness was legendary, and I remember rows with my mother, and wondering why we needed to visit them at all. When we did so, I remember my parents getting drunk while Julian and I tried to play with their daughter Danielle.

Maureen Lynch, wife of the Taoiseach, was another dear friend of the family; Jack Lynch was my godfather. As small boys wearing velvet suits we were presented to Princess Grace of Monaco, who was patron of the Dublin Theatre Festival, and we met the Queen of Spain.

Godfrey Quigley, a leading actor at the time, stayed with us while he recuperated from a broken leg. He was a weighty man with a beautiful booming voice, and he loved placing a bet. One afternoon as we watched the racing with him he got so excited that, instead of resting his plastered leg on a stool, he banged it loudly on the ground as he egged his horse on.

If our theatrical home life was different from that of my friends – and I was starting to learn that it was – I had the utter good fortune to make friends with Matthew, and to spend time in his house, which was across the road from ours. I was welcomed by his parents, Con and Oriana, and I became a surrogate sibling for Matthew, who was an only child at the time. Clearly, his parents believed that Matthew would gain from the friendship, but I think I was the one who benefitted the most.

Oriana was from the Ascendancy class – she was a descendant of the Duke of Wellington. She was tall, thin and very beautiful, with fair hair which she kept long and girlish well into her seventies.

Spending time with them, I saw a family whose work did not dominate their lives. Oriana loved talking to us. She would listen closely to tales of our adventures, drawing us out. She would praise us when we completed projects like building a go-kart, without drawing attention to the fact that Matthew's gentle father Con had been a pivotal guide. I adored her, and viewed her as my second mother. And Con modelled a different kind of maleness to my father's very studied, assertive and feisty personality. Con spent time with Matthew and me and enjoyed his family life, instead of seeming to pour all his energies into his work.

The couple was curious and engaged, and always hugely supportive to us children. I couldn't help comparing my family to Matthew's – it was unavoidable – and it was clear to me that his, without doubt, was better than mine.

In the summers I was invited to Con's original family home, Manch Farm in West Cork. I'd spend several weeks there, and it was a haven, like walking into an Enid Blyton adventure. Matthew's grandfather, a retired judge, presided there and we spent many sunny afternoons playing croquet with him on the lawn opposite the house.

We also helped with the haymaking. We were allowed to drive the tractor which was a big thrill, and we helped to bring the harvest in, working as best we could and empowered by being physically at one with the men. When we were tired and hungry after a morning's physical work, the sight of Oriana bumping through the field in her jeep was more welcome than I can say. Downing tools, we'd run over to her and help lift rugs and baskets out of the boot. And we'd watch as she unpacked these, producing a picnic fit for a film set. There would be lemonade to wash everything down and, always, sweets at the end.

Far from being grand the house, which dated from the 1700s, could best be described as ramshackle. There had been a fire, and the staircase of the main turret was burnt, making only parts of the house habitable. Matthew and I yearned to sleep in the tower, and initially were met with a firm 'No'. But we were persistent and, eventually, after Con and Oriana had checked the tower out and declared it safe, they gave in.

'But boys, we're trusting you,' said Con. 'There are to be no high jinks. You've got to be responsible for one another.'

Jumping up and down with excitement, we stocked up on crisps and biscuits, then crossed the ladder that bridged the gap between the main house and the burnt-out staircase that led to the tower. And after a wonderfully illicit midnight feast, we settled there to sleep in camp beds. Those glorious summers added such richness to my life.

Three

Coming of Age

I was still getting some acting work, and not just in advertisements; there were some minor roles in the theatre too. And in 1971, when I was thirteen, I was offered a small part in the remake of the film *Black Beauty*, which starred Mark Lester of *Oliver!* fame as Joe. It was an English production, and was filmed on location in Co. Wicklow. There were long days with a lot of sitting around, but jeez, it was way better than school.

I played a farm hand who comes across Black Beauty towards the end of the horse's life. He'd had his glory days and was tired. The farmer who owned him was old, grumpy and bad-tempered. He wanted the horse to work, but I loved Black Beauty, and wanted to make life easier for him. In one scene, when he told me to move the horse I wasn't working quickly enough, and when the farmer came to get him he was angry, because I hadn't got the job started.

In the scene he says angrily, 'Don't be messing with the horse,' and he slaps me across the face. At least it's made to look as if he does so, but the actor playing the farmer was old and finding it difficult to coordinate the fake slap. We spent twenty minutes trying to get the shot to look genuine.

Eventually, the director came up to me and said, 'Can I have a word with you?'

I was taken aback. The director wanted a word with *me*? That was unprecedented.

'I'm a little bit uncomfortable about this,' he said, 'but I'll ask you anyway.' He stroked his chin meditatively. 'It would be really great if we could get this scene shot, but we're not getting it.' He then took a fifty-pound note out of his pocket and fingered it. Looking around surreptitiously, he murmured, 'If I gave you this, would you mind if we give you just one good slap?'

Agreeing with a grin, I pocketed the proffered note. The slap, when it came, almost floored me, but thankfully we got the scene in that single take.

'Are you okay?' asked the director, seeing me rub my reddened cheek. I nodded. This to me was just part of the stimulation and excitement of performing. And it suited me. It felt natural and entirely comfortable. Through such experiences I began to understand the adult world some-what, and in doing so gained a window into my father's theatrical world. And, gaining awareness of his status and achievements I became proud of him, proud of being his son and delighting in the association.

I continued to attend my classes at the Brendan Smith Academy each Saturday, and I adored it, as much for the friends I made as for the acting. Whiling away the minutes before our class began, we'd gather outside on the steps, which provided a good opportunity for us to practise our flirting skills.

We were a precocious bunch. I can't remember the name of the first girl who caught my fancy, but I remember exactly what she looked like. She had fair, very curly hair. The only difficult thing was that I was a tiny bit shorter than she was. I suspected this was always going to be a problem for us. I made sure to sit down quickly, so that the height difference wouldn't be apparent; or, if we were standing, I'd make sure that I was on a lower step, and then there was no issue. We could complicitly pretend it was the step that caused this differential.

The chats were great, but we never took it further than flirting. There were no fumbles. No kisses either – I think both of us would have been terrified if there had been. This was just practice.

And then, working on a film, I fell in love. *And No One Could Save Her*, released in 1973, was a corny, typically Irish-American piece about a woman who is searching for her husband. The last she heard of him he was boarding a plane for Ireland, so she arrives in hot pursuit.

The woman was played by the American film star Lee Remick, and I fell for her hook, line and sinker. I had a small part in the film, with little dialogue, but I appeared in a great many scenes and was called to the set most days.

I'd arrive early for make-up and costume, and then I'd sit on the bus being royally fed, hoping for just a glance of Lee. When I encountered her my pulse would quicken, and when she smiled and stopped to say a few words, my day was made! I'd lie in bed at night going through the encounter, imagining scenarios in which the age barrier didn't exist. A journalist came to the set one day and asked me what I thought of the star. I don't know what my mumbled reply actually was, but I was quoted as saying, 'She is very charming.'

And if Lee Remick was charming to me – and of course she was – it was the actor Milo O'Shea who really looked out for me. He played a bumbling lawyer called Patrick Dooley and I was 'O'Toole', his clerk and runner. I'm not sure if my mother, a good friend of his, had asked him to keep an eye on me, but he certainly did. He was generous and kind, making sure I was always comfortable in this adult world. I learned a lot from him.

The following year I played a boy in a teenage gang in a film called *A Quiet Day in Belfast*. In the film, we got ourselves into various entanglements with rivals. It was fun, I loved acting. It seemed miraculous that I was given money for doing something I enjoyed so much.

Back in school I was the envy of many of my friends, and became 'the bank in class'. If anybody was short of money it was, 'Ronan, would you give me a loan? I want to buy something,' and I'd say, 'Oh, all right.' Acting and earning money made me extremely popular.

Life wasn't all about films. There was my education to consider as well. I attended St Conleth's College, a small private Catholic school for boys on Dublin's Clyde Road. There was an extraordinary mix of teachers there: some were inspiring; others, like the French teacher Mr Freutren, were extreme disciplinarians. When the Germans invaded France during World War II they promised any Breton who chose to fight with them that once France was under German rule, Brittany would remain independent. Accepting this pledge, the French teacher fought alongside the Germans for the Nazi cause. The man was a Nazi! He scared the bejaysus out of all of us.

I had many friends there and I'd known some of them since primary school. One of them was Philip Lee, who became a lifelong friend. I spent so much time at his house, and it wasn't only because I liked his company; I loved his mother Denise. She was so kind to me, and so wise. It was as if I was her fourth son.

Philip and I took up fencing together, taking the sport extremely seriously, and through our participation in various tournaments we built up a friendly rivalry.

There was a small girls' school in the vicinity called Miss Meredith's. It had a superb reputation, but was lacking in some areas, so some of the more academic girls needed better maths and science teaching than the school could provide. It was arranged that they could come up to St Conleth's to attend classes with us. I felt very comfortable in their presence, I had no hidden agenda. I really enjoyed them as people, preferring them in many ways to boys. I made many female friends.

Coming up to the Leaving Certificate, I wasn't sure what I wanted to do next. As a younger teenager I'd thought of studying Veterinary Medicine – I'd always loved animals and had adored my life at Manch Farm – but by the age of seventeen I'd gone off the idea. Living in Dublin, I was more comfortable with something that felt more present. Julian had embarked on a business degree with a view to working in marketing, and the parents of my friends tended to be lawyers, bankers and doctors; the ethos of those professions seemed to fit better with city living.

I decided to take aptitude tests and ping, up at the top was law. I thought I'd be okay with that, it was a good notion. I mentioned this to Philip, and when he said he planned to study law that clinched it! If I had him for company we'd have some fun. And, starting together at University College Dublin (UCD) in 1975, we did!

I was a good student and law came easily to me. I was interested in the logic of it, and the follow-through; I enjoyed the intellectual rigour of arguing things out. In our spare time Philip and I carried on with our fencing, training every day. By this time both of us were pretty proficient: we represented Ireland twice, in the European Junior Championships in London and the World Junior Championships in Vienna. We were nicknamed 'Bill and Ben the fencing men'.

I deliberately avoided the college's theatre society – known as DramSoc – for the first couple of years, because I wanted to give other things a chance to take my fancy. Besides, I'd gone to see one or two shows and I didn't think much of them. College productions can sometimes be driven more by enthusiasm than by true talent.

Much as I enjoyed the intellectual side of my course, by Third Year I had started to realise that, as a profession, law was not for me. I decided to continue with the process, which involved getting my degree in tandem with the Law Society exams, but I was pretty sure I wouldn't end up as a professional lawyer.

I'd begun to realise, somewhat belatedly, that acting was in my blood. I missed it. In Second Year, I'd befriended Martin Drury. He lived on Herbert Park, near my old school. We'd met now and then before we started college, but at UCD we became close. He was interested in drama, and he persuaded me to join DramSoc that year. I went to an audition session in LG1 – the basement room where the plays were rehearsed and performed – and found there a varied crew, some of whom spent their entire days and evenings in LG1.

There were a number of very deeply committed aspiring thespians who put themselves forward as directors of the productions that they wanted to stage. Some of the plays were dramatic classics, some were wacky and experimental; many were in between.

Besides Martin Drury, I learned a lot from another student, Ben Barnes, who later became Artistic Director at the Abbey Theatre. Martin was keen to direct; we put a few projects forward and we performed a couple of lunchtime shows together. Martin is an extremely rigorous and conscientious person, and performing with him proved an intense experience. We were experimenting, and it was tough – it felt a bit like cutting teeth. I loved the opportunity to try out very different styles of theatre, and it confirmed my growing notion that the theatrical life was a far more powerful instinct for me than practising law.

In Fourth Year, the system at the time for law students was that we get an apprenticeship in a law firm, and our parents had to stump up the fee. I had the bizarre experience of serving the solicitor's apprenticeship in a barely furnished attic office up above the main workspace. I was shown the room, directed towards a desk and a chair, and I sat there waiting for someone to show me what to do. I waited, and waited. Soon it became clear that nobody was going to give me any tasks, or none that were meaningful.

Sometimes, sitting there twiddling my thumbs, I imagined myself in a Dickens novel, because apprenticeships, it seemed, had little changed since he had penned his classics. My parents had paid a fat fee, expecting me to be readied for a legal career, but that didn't happen.

Sitting alone, looking at the phone that never rang, I decided my role wasn't that of an apprentice at all. I was the office runner. Bored, I ended up rather guiltily reading the romantic correspondence between the last incumbent and the woman he dated. He was the son of the solicitor I worked for and had left the letters in the desk drawer. The whole thing was a charade, but I thought I'd better finish it, simply because my parents were paying and I didn't want to let them down.

I duly qualified. I had my third-level law degree and gained the parchment as proof. Having thus salved my conscience by dutifully finishing off the professional qualification as a solicitor, I turned my back on it all, ran away with the circus, and went acting instead.

Four

Treading the Boards

Shortly after I qualified as a solicitor I moved out of home. This mystified my parents.

'You're leaving?' Putting down *The Irish Times*, my father peered at me, and my mother put her cup down with a bang, slopping coffee into the saucer.

'Why?' My father looked shell-shocked. 'What have we done wrong?'

'You haven't done anything wrong.'

He'd pushed his glasses onto the top of his head, and was staring at me quizzically. Neither of them could understand what could make me leave this large, comfortable, free and, most importantly, conveniently situated house.

'I want to grow up,' I said, and when they realised I had made up my mind, they let me be. Philip Lee and I joined a flatshare in Churchtown, on the south side of Dublin City. It worked out well. Having known each other for so many years, it was nice starting out on this new adventure together. Philip, making use of his law degree, started an apprenticeship, and I began to tread the boards.

While I was enjoying life and relishing the freedom, Philip sometimes felt frustrated. He was bored with his apprenticeship. It didn't help that Ed, who took the third room in the flat, had an altogether more exciting life than Philip did. Ed was a male model, and a series of long-legged girls regularly arrived with him to the flat and accompanied him to his room.

'How does he do it?' Philip muttered, as we tried to ignore the enthusiastic bedroom noises.

I laughed. I did, to some extent, share his jealousy, but unlike the day-to-day drudgery he endured my working life was, potentially at least, full of glamour and fun.

But the two of us did occasionally score. If I came back to the flat to find the flap to the gas meter open, I knew that meant Philip had a hot date and I was to skedaddle, and he did the same for me. In fact, the smell of cooking trout was another giveaway. It was Philip's signature dish – in other words the only one he had mastered.

I don't know how the girls put up with the Arctic conditions, because the flat was freezing. In the winter, we'd wake to find ice on the inside of the windows. We'd wear hats and gloves in bed in an effort to ward off the cold.

My career started slowly, and that was hard. I wasn't any good at doing nothing, so it was a relief when, after a while, I was more often in work than out of it.

I performed on theatre tours around Ireland, and occasionally I toured abroad. I was aware that I was lucky. I knew that my parents' connections, as well as my childhood acting experience, had helped to get me to this busy, fulfilling place. There were Bernard Farrell comedies in the Abbey, there was *A Christmas Carol* in the Gate.

I simply loved acting. It's fantastic. What I enjoyed about it was the tension of delivery. You've learned the part, but when you go out on the stage it's all-consuming; it's exhilarating. And although I enjoyed my film and television work I much preferred the stage because, when you are literally treading the boards, you are more in the moment.

Early in 1979, I had a part in the film *SOS Titanic* in Shepperton Studios near London, directed by Bill Hale. That experience – with filming also on location in the Waldorf Hotel and on the Isle of Man – was an eye opener. There were long days of filming, but on many of those days I was never called.

Friends from Dublin, Gerard McSorley and Philip O'Sullivan, also had parts in the film. The three of us would arrive together at the studio and would, more often than not, be told to sit quietly for the day. On one of the days when we did have work, on the supposed 'ship', there were a lot of extras involved. Whenever the director shouted 'Action!' they all ran towards the flooded, wet side of the ship. The rest of us watched them, wondering what on earth they thought they were doing.

'I don't understand it,' I said. 'Why would you want to get wet?'

It turned out that the extras had a clause in their contracts known as 'wet money'. In other words, if they got wet performing their scenes, they were given extra. Now it made sense!

Although there were some memorable moments, when I was praised for my work, or when I was shot for a close-up and felt that familiar adrenaline rush, there was too much time to think and to give voice to all my insecurities. Was I good enough? Would I make it as an actor?

Yet even after a good day I wouldn't always be satisfied. Acting seemed too easy. I was earning a great deal of money and yet the work wasn't challenging. Again I had the realisation that film can be very hit and miss, and you don't get the same buzz from it as you do in theatre.

Living in London for that time was, undoubtedly, good for me. Although I missed Ireland and my real friends, it was good being thrown in with the cast, learning to fit in and make new friends. I did a lot of growing up there.

Back home, there were times when I found myself 'resting', but from 1980 onwards my father made sure that I was never short of meaningful employment. He set me to work with him in his office. My father's main job was to manage the Olympia Theatre in Dame Street, while also working on the Dublin Theatre Festival, however, his office was at the Brendan Smith Theatre Academy in nearby George's Street.

I wasn't a very gracious employee. I felt I was being forced to work. It bothered me that my father assumed that I would be happy to follow in his career footsteps, because I wasn't at all sure that that was what I wanted. Besides, there wasn't a lot of work for me to do. Was this just my father's way of proving he had a dutiful son? In time, I put my objections to one side and settled in. And that's when I began to find the work rewarding.

It was a chance to get to know my father, something I had so yearned to do when I was a child. And in getting to know him I began to view his strengths, and his weaknesses. I had always been aware that my father was larger than life – it was simply his character – but I hadn't realised that his eccentricities were noticed and remarked upon by others.

It turned out that my father had quite a few nicknames. And though his close staff made sure not to bombard me with these, I couldn't help becoming aware of them through overhearing office banter. I wasn't sure why they called him Bungie – but when I heard him referred to as Captain Mainwaring I laughed out loud.

This character, played by Arthur Lowe in the BBC comedy series *Dad's Army*, not only bore a physical resemblance to my father, but Dad had also adopted that same clipped delivery over the years – especially when he was barking out instructions at speed. I'd loved the programme as a child and had always sensed the likeness. The nickname was utterly appropriate.

My laughter, however, was tinged with an uneasy guilt, because my father's frequent indignation and tendency to drift into pomposity often made me cringe. More embarrassing still were the times he fabricated temper tantrums. He had a habit of jumping up and down on his hat in airports, or other public places, in order to get special attention.

But if he was stubborn, he was also highly driven. He was a natural leader – a natural risk-taker too – and he had considerable persuasive powers. That was fortunate, as he had to generate enthusiasm in others if his plans were to be realised. There was something of the American showman Barnum about him.

Being a bit of a workaholic, my father often ate his lunch at his desk. But rather than send out for sandwiches, he would order from the Connacht Restaurant on Dame Court. A waitress would appear, smartly dressed in her traditional uniform of a black skirt and white blouse, and would ceremoniously place his lunch tray on the table in front of him.

He loved the social side of the theatre, and was known to be the very best company. Back in the 1950s, he wrote and produced a number of successful comedies that played in Dublin and around the country. There was no doubt that he had great status, and that he commanded the respect of his colleagues through his history of interaction in many roles in the Irish theatre and arts worlds.

These had led to his honorary doctorate from the National University of Ireland; his awards from the French government for collaborative theatre projects with French theatre companies; and his appointment to the Censorship Appeal Board. But what I witnessed now above all these honours was his terrifyingly obdurate stubbornness and drive.

He would relax during a night out. And if, after a few drinks in the Olympia and maybe dinner at Trocadero restaurant, the excesses of the night left my father exceptionally drunk, he was easy enough to handle. When he went too far, he had a tendency to mutter, 'Poor Brennie,' and when I heard those words I knew it was time to get him a taxi. That happened a few times, but it wasn't a problem.

I imagined that this eccentricity was part of my father's make-up, the way he had always been, but my mother expressed her concerns. She had long been confiding in me, and many times over the years had let me know of my parents' sometimes stormy relationship. She often complained that he wasn't talking to her. But now she would say that she feared my father was losing his grip a little.

'It's just the drink,' I'd say, hoping this was true.

'No, Ronan. Something's not right,' she said. 'Can you please watch him carefully?'

I promised to report back. Did I realise, back then, that she was right? And that there was, indeed, something wrong with my father? Could I see that his bluster, and determination to stay in control at all times, was more than his normal eccentricity, and was becoming more extreme? I don't know, although I can see it now in hindsight. And though I could see that he got his colleagues to attend to as many details as they could, I wasn't aware that he was bluffing because *he* was aware of his increasing incompetence. It simply didn't occur to me.

But if I couldn't see this clearly, having never seen my father at work before, his colleagues and staff had become well aware of it. They begged him to take time off. That was like a red rag to a bull. He refused point blank, and held on to his role with a ferocious tenacity – a remarkable achievement, if a misjudged one.

Although my theatre work was plentiful, it was becoming less rewarding. In parallel with working with my father in his office when not acting, a slow realisation was dawning on me that comedic wimps or shy, sensitive souls seemed to be perceived by directors to be my strong card as an actor. This was undeniable: playing such characters always got me laughs.

My mother wasn't keen on my 'wimp roles', and she made her distaste abundantly clear. She'd berate me about it, telling me how in her career, which included musicals, there'd always been a really good variety. Sometimes, she'd be overheard berating me in the bar after the show. I got ribbed about it. But I was used to being teased when we all gathered for after-show drinks. I'd be ridiculed for having just one pint of Guinness when most of the cast had many.

Those were good times, meeting a great range and type of people. And though, despite my mother's low opinion, I could have gone on indefinitely playing all the wimp characters that were given to me, I was rigorous, and determined not to simply drift. It would have been a waste of time. Being typecast simply didn't suit me.

I decided to take a break to reconsider my future, and took off on the J1 visa scheme to the US over the summer of 1980, to 'find myself' as the phrase went at the time. I wasn't seeking any acting work there, I just wanted to step back from career issues and, travelling from west to east, took casual employment to keep myself in funds. This was possibly an act of unconscious self-protection, and when I calmed down somewhat over the month and a half I spent in America, I returned home with a clearer head.

When I walked through the arrival doors at Dublin Airport, I was astonished to see my father waiting for me. I stared at him in total disbelief. He hadn't told me he was coming, and this was truly unprecedented behaviour. He had taken time off work to stand in the airport waiting, so that he could welcome me home – and I realised immediately what a significant signal this was.

While I felt surprise and pleasure, I also felt uncomfortable as I absorbed the reality that there was more than an element of the 'Prodigal Son' story about this for him. He had missed me. *Really* missed me, and had been terrified that I'd gone for good. This was an extraordinary revelation.

I also sensed a nascent insecurity in him that I had never seen before. This, in its turn, made me feel strangely insecure. It was a signal of vulnerability that didn't chime with my experience of him, of my image of him as an indefatigable fighter, a 'Trojan'.

'Hello son,' he said. 'Welcome home.' We shook hands firmly (there were no hugs) and smiled.

'Thanks,' I said, 'and thanks for coming out to pick me up.'

There was a short silence, which I broke. 'So how are things for you?' I asked.

'Busy. Busy. That time of year, you know. Festival approaching. It's good to have you back.'

We chatted in the car going home, but he didn't ask me about my experience in America, preferring the safety of theatre talk. He told me how things were with the Olympia, with the Dublin Theatre Festival, with the Academy – all the comfortable and known territory of the dominant world of work. And the very next day there I was, back in the office, behind the metaphoric shop counter, apron on, preparing for my immediate next role of Box Office Manager for that year's Dublin Theatre Festival.

The job itself did not float my boat particularly, but the people around it were lively and engaging. Michael Colgan was Festival Manager at the time (my father was Festival Director), and his forceful, energetic personality created a spirited, somewhat charged, atmosphere.

After seeing this seasonal work through, there was then an exotic trip to Hong Kong with my father's production of *Romeo and Juliet*, and he was assiduously courting me to come on board with his activities. The origins of this very unlikely touring destination were that an aged Jesuit teacher from my father's school years in Belvedere College was still actively, and somewhat unbelievably, teaching. This was in Hong Kong. Many of his Chinese ex-pupils were now part of the civil service work force, and some were senior civil servants. These particular civil servants were then persuaded (or, perhaps more accurately, instructed) by him to invite an Irish theatre company to perform at their arts festival. Given that there was a pattern of English companies doing so, why not an Irish company as well? The tour was planned, the show rehearsed, and off we flew.

This saw the start of some acting careers as well as charting progress for some romantic liaisons – or of one in particular. Malcolm Douglas played Romeo to Kate Thompson's Juliet. Their performances were glittering, with a wonderful chemistry between them – helped by the fact, obvious to all the cast, that off stage the two of them were as besotted with each other as were the characters they played.

When Malcolm and Kate were busy rehearsing, the rest of us had a great deal more freedom to enjoy all that Hong Kong had to offer. In the main, this was highly enjoyable, but one night I found it all a bit too much. There was a night out after one performance on this trip when most of the company, including my father and me, went to a night-club in downtown Kowloon.

A group of young Chinese women who were there were being particularly friendly and hospitable towards us. Fairly quickly and in a breezy, business-like way, they made it clear they were ladies of the night, ready to sell their wares. Their proposals came as quite a surprise to me, young innocent abroad that I was. The fun-seeking actors and some of the off-stage crew from the show, including my father, were engaging in this conversation in a jocular manner, with lots of banter and laughter.

One of the women seemed fascinated by the fact that my father was wearing two watches. She asked him why, a question I'm sure others had wondered. Holding out his hand to display his wrist, he explained that they were set at two different times.

'This one is on Irish time,' he said, pointing to the one he always wore, 'and this one, this is on Hong Kong time.'

I felt uneasy at the way the girl had singled my father out and, having watched from the sidelines for a minute or two, I said my farewells and made a hurried, and frankly somewhat panicked, exit back to the hotel. I didn't want to see, or ever even know of, my father's involvement in such shenanigans. I was tense when we met for a late breakfast the following day but, making no reference to the night before, we simply talked about the coming day. We never did talk about that night, much to my relief.

Five

My Father Deteriorates

On my return home, as my twenty-third birthday approached, I continued to work as an actor. But I also took on an occasional directing and producing role, so I stopped working for my father. Therefore, I didn't see first-hand the signs that his powers were slowly failing or that, despite his best efforts, deficiencies, which he had initially hidden, were now revealing themselves. Nevertheless, I was made fully aware of them. His colleagues and employees made sure of that. They rang me frequently to report on his condition.

'There's definitely something wrong here,' his assistant said. 'Brendan is having considerable difficulty keeping pace with the work. And he's getting worse.'

'How does this manifest?' I asked, my heart sinking.

'He's getting behind with his correspondence, and I have to continually remind him to do it. That's out of character.'

'Yes, you're right,' I said with a sigh. My father always prided himself on keeping on top of things.

'And when I hassle him, he just bluffs and says, "Oh, I'm sure you can deal with that." And of course I can, and do, out of necessity.'

'Does he write *any* of his own letters?' I asked.

'Oh, he tries. He came in on Monday and, when I reminded him, sat down to write letters at once. But when I looked in on him two hours later, he'd only written one paragraph. So of course I had to take over. But Ronan, it's worrying.'

He was right. It *was* worrying, not least because he was still not admitting that there was anything wrong. But the effort of hiding whatever was wrong with him was causing him increased stress, which no doubt hastened his decline. And there did seem to be a speeding up of his decline; it was like watching a runaway train.

I was on tour, acting in Wexford around this time, and my parents decided to pay me a visit. When I met them after the show, my mother was in a terrible state. Forgetting to congratulate me, or comment in any way on my performance, she launched into a tirade on my father.

'He almost killed us on the journey down,' she said, explaining that he had pulled out to overtake, and narrowly missed hitting an oncoming car. Her hand shook as she puffed on her cigarette, and she was unusually subdued. And my father? He tried to brush it off, insisting that she was overreacting.

None of us mentioned his deteriorating health. My father, I believe, still thought he'd managed to keep it secret and, in truth, we all had passively participated in this pattern of denial. I suppose we couldn't face our fears, and we continued to avoid facing it for months, while the incidences steadily accumulated.

At around this time, when the Dublin Theatre Festival was approaching, Michael Colgan rang. 'I need you to come in and talk to me,' he said, 'but not in the office.'

'That sounds ominous,' I thought, as I made my way to the meeting. We had a good, frank talk. Michael started the meeting by saying, 'Ronan, I think there is something very wrong with your father.' And I had to agree, 'Yeah, I think I know that.'

'You do?'

I nodded.

'Look, Ronan. I like your father, and I respect him a great deal. Well,' he continued, pushing his glasses up, 'we all do. I mean, he founded the Theatre Festival – he's a legend. But Ronan, he's becoming a liability – a loose cannon.'

'Oh.' This was worse than I had feared.

'We need to find ways to protect him, because otherwise he could make serious mistakes and, as his number two, I could be held responsible, and be in the line of fire.'

'Yes, I do see that.'

'Good. Because I can't sit around and watch a crisis happen. And this is where you come in.'

I sighed, thinking, I know where this is going! 'You want me to keep an eye on him?'

'Exactly! Could you please do that? And act as a buffer? I'd hate his reputation to be besmirched.'

I left that meeting with a mix of emotions. Although I was glad it was now out in the open, I worried terribly about how exactly I could manage my father. But I did everything possible to lighten his load. Any time I could, I helped out in the George's Street office. This was tough when I had acting jobs on, but I just did it. I became like my father's assistant: I could, so I did. It felt entirely natural.

I was at a party one night, chatting to a guy I hadn't met before. He was a businessman of some sort and was interested in the theatre and quizzing me on my role in it. I gave him a rundown and, looking at me with wide eyes, he said, 'I thought *I* worked hard. But you must never stop.' I couldn't deny it. It was the truth.

And then my father said he was off to Paris. My mother rang me, in a state.

'Ronan, can you dissuade him from this trip?' she said. 'It's madness. Can you just tell him he mustn't go?'

'I can try,' I said, and I did, but to no avail.

'I have meetings over there,' he said, muttering that he knew my mother had put me up to this. 'Important meetings. And besides, I deserve a break now the festival is over.' He seemed determined to push the boat out and prove that he was capable of the trip.

He rang from Paris the first evening to say that he had arrived safely. My mother relaxed. He contacted her again the following evening, but then the calls stopped. There was nothing from him at all for two very long days. He had, to all intents and purposes, simply disappeared.

'I take it you've rung the hotel,' I said when she phoned, sounding utterly distraught.

'Well of course I have,' she said. 'His clothes are still in his room, but the management hasn't seen or heard from him either.'

The last sighting of him was when he had left a restaurant where a group of them was enjoying a night out. For once, I felt my mother's histrionics were entirely justified.

When she rang to tell me that he was safe, I was both relieved and worried. Rather than prove he was capable of the trip, my father had confirmed all my mother's, and my own, worst fears: he could no longer enjoy his independence. And he would *hate* that.

A doctor from a hospital in Paris had contacted my mother to say that my father had fallen on the pavement and hit his head. He was badly bruised and, to the hospital's eyes, strangely disorientated.

'The doctor assumed his confusion was a result of the bang on the head he got when he fell,' my mother explained. 'They carried out a battery of tests, and it took them two days to extract his name and contact details.'

That news was bad enough. But when he got home, bruised but unrepentant, it turned out that he had been the victim of a scam as well. His credit card had been used to pay the bill for the party of colleagues he was with that evening; a smooth and practised con was used in which the card was taken from him for payment, but in fact also paid for a series of rapid visits to a number of neighbouring bars, chalking up a tidy sum of bogus charges.

The scam was eventually proven and the matter closed, but the incident highlighted the extent of his vulnerability. The whole debacle made my mother and me painfully aware that there was a very real health problem of some kind at play.

But still my father blustered, insisting that both the fall and the scam could have happened to anyone. It was clear that he had to hide the reality of his illness. And he kept this up week on week, month on month, and year on year. He surely should have known that this plan had no chance of ultimate success?

The truth was that he couldn't bear the thought of a life without his work. It was unimaginable to him, because his work in the world of theatre was what defined him, what made him the person he was. He could not contemplate being anyone other than that person. Another explanation was that he was already so advanced in his symptoms that his reasoning had, in effect, left him already.

After the bungled trip to Paris my mother's concern grew in intensity, as did my father's illness. She gave me constant and detailed updates on his difficulties coping at home, as well as at work. I was drawn in closer and closer to the rising crisis, and it was impossible now to ignore it.

My father had asked me to become part-time Company Secretary and Board Director for the Olympia Theatre. I'd been resisting it, but now accepted his offer, seeing it as a way I could help out as well as observe exactly how he was performing. After all, I reasoned, if I wanted to spend any substantial time with my father, I had to work with him.

In October 1984 I met my mother for a spot of lunch. She seemed particularly agitated, and when we got to the coffee stage she began, 'Your father's mother.'

'Yes?'

'She went a little bit funny you know.' Pointing at her head, she made a face.

'A bit funny? You mean ...'

'She had premature senility.'

'Really? No, I didn't know that.'

I sighed, noticing my mother's eyes jumping with fear. This was the last thing I wanted to hear, and I'm not sure I absorbed the information. It was easier to imagine that my father was suffering from some kind of depression, and that this was what caused his absent-mindedness. I told myself that this was just my mother being a bit melodramatic. She was, after all, inclined to be anxious and overwrought about things. I should have taken this information seriously, and in fact should have acted on it – or helped my mother to do so – but instead I found myself reassuring her.

Was I, like my father, in denial? Was it just that I didn't want this problem right now? Because that was the case. I had other things on my mind: better, more exciting things. TEAM Theatre (a theatre-in-education company) was looking for a new Artistic Director. The outgoing Director Martin Drury, the college friend who had introduced me to DramSoc, had approached me, wondering if I would be interested in becoming his successor. 'Would you like to apply?' he asked me.

TEAM Educational Theatre was a long-established, well-regarded company that toured schools and youth clubs with a team of six actors, performing commissioned plays with issues and themes that were of relevance to young people.

Back in 1983 I had acted in a play for the company, *Then Moses Met Marconi*, written by comedy playwright Bernard Farrell. The plot revolved around a young journalist who returned to her home town in rural Ireland and took a job in the local pirate radio station. She had radical ideas for the time and wanted to bring feminism to the fore, but her boss opposed her at every turn. I played Justin Day, the janitor, who ends up stepping in as an unlikely presenter. It's a comedy with serious overtones.

To prepare for the play, we spent a couple of months in the Tyrone Guthrie Centre at Annaghmakerrig in Co. Monaghan. The actor, Tyrone Guthrie, had lived in this wonderful house with its lake and acres of woodland, and on his death in 1971, he bequeathed it to the Irish State to be used as a residential facility for creative artists. It had been open for a year by the time we stayed there, in the winter of 1982.

Martin Drury led the retreat to the centre. The process was that the cast of seven worked in the retreat's performance room, essentially playing games and working up a sense of camaraderie.

Bernard Farrell submitted a draft script, and he observed many of the improvisation sessions; in this way we had a real input into the finished script. It was a truly wonderful experience, and a bonding one too. In the evenings we gathered for dinner with the other artists in residence – writers, musicians and visual artists – and ate dinner together every night with the director of the centre, Bernard Loughlin. The retreat, in such beautiful surroundings, was a wonderful vehicle, not just for the sake of the play, but for uniting the cast. It all added up to a pleasant and vivacious working environment.

We took the play round the country at the start of 1983, playing to secondary and vocational schools, and had a very positive reaction from the students. I was proud to be part of such an innovative production and enjoyed playing Justin Day; it was an interesting part, allowing me to display a full range of emotions.

Julian Erskine, a man who was to become important later in my life, was the lighting designer on the production. He had worked for my father in the Dublin Theatre Festival and had become a friend. He toured with us and attended a good few performances.

He continually told me how much my performance had moved him. 'It gets to me every time,' he said. 'You recite that poignant speech – I know it's coming; I know what you'll say, but each time the power of it just takes my breath away.'

53

And there *was* something special about that play; it felt important, and the message was strong. It showed that local opinion and concerns got brushed under the carpet back then – particularly female concerns – and it caused great debate among the students.

I'd loved the integrity of the company and how everyone involved was working with the same aims in mind, and I was eager to be further involved. I duly applied for the position of Director and was delighted when my application was successful.

My father was not impressed. In fact, he was perturbed. 'What did you accept *that* for?' he asked, disdain in his voice. 'That's not *real* theatre.'

'What do you mean it's not real theatre? We perform *real* plays.'

'Yes, to schools! Taking the play around in a van.'

My father was very set in his ways, and believed that *real* theatre could only take place in theatres. I tried to explain to him that TEAM was *very* real theatre. It was also very purposeful, indeed often challenging, but equally often deeply and immediately rewarding in a way that mainstream theatre frequently isn't. But still he raised his eyebrows, showing complete bafflement.

But that's where my father and I differed. For him, theatre was partly about the glory: the personalities; the recognition; the glitz of the first night; whereas to me it's always been more about the greater good. And anyway, it's not as if I'd turned my back on 'real' theatre. At this time, alongside my dual roles with TEAM and the Olympia, I was also acting in the Abbey, Peacock and Gate theatres regularly for short seasons. Maintaining this crazy work schedule was dysfunctional behaviour, and the excitement of it all was the drug that fuelled the dysfunction.

Perhaps I should have taken on the unasked-for advice proffered by Michael Colgan, the larger-than-life director of the Gate Theatre. Watching me flit between theatre production and acting, he said to me one day, 'Ronan, one of these days, you'll have to choose.'

'Choose?' I had no idea what he was talking about.

'Yes. You can aim to be an actor of the calibre of John Kavanagh, or you can aim to be me.'

This made me laugh at the time, but perhaps he had a point. Maybe it was time now to concentrate on this other facet of theatre.

Six

Juggling

We all struggled on. Then, on 26 June 1985, my father received a most prestigious award. The French Embassy gave him an honorary upgrade award as Commandeur de L'Ordre des Arts et des Lettres, in recognition for all the French theatre companies he had brought to the Dublin Theatre Festival over many years. All of the colleagues he had worked with received an invitation to this most glittering event.

The French Embassy oozes grandeur, and it truly was a cheery and celebratory event. Nobody observing my father that evening would have guessed the state of his befuddled mind and, when the ambassador, delivering his eulogy in awkward English said, 'You love the world of theatre in which you have spent yourself,' he cannot have known the insightfulness of his remark. Because spent he surely was. But as the audience clapped and cheered, including those who had to increasingly cover for my father, the phrase rang around my head, and I felt hurt for him.

It was now taking my father two hours to simply get out of the house, but he still insisted on travelling to his precious work. As for me, I had to do what had to be done. And that meant getting into the office early, because my father wasn't getting there until midday. And at this stage, he was still driving.

My father had a space at the office where he parked every day, up against the wall. One afternoon, having said 'Goodbye', he headed for his car to drive home. Five minutes later, he appeared back in the office.

'Have you forgotten something?' He didn't answer and, turning around, I noticed that he was badly shaken. 'What is it?' I asked.

'I seem to have crashed the car.'

Shamefaced, he led me down to the car park, and the damage was worse than I could have imagined. The whole bonnet had concertinaed. 'What happened, Dad?'

'I don't know.' He looked at me and shrugged, his face a picture of confusion. 'I turned on the engine and the car leapt forwards. I think there's something wrong with it.'

'I don't think so, Dad,' I said. 'You must have left the car in drive – and maybe left off the handbrake?'

His gaze hardened. 'Well,' he said. 'Anyone can make that mistake.'

Relieved that nobody had been injured, I insisted that his driving would have to stop. He didn't like the decision and mentioned his opposition to it to everyone, colleagues and family alike. But they all concurred with my advice. My mother expressed deep relief, saying she'd been worried for months that he would kill either himself or someone else. We both agreed we had got away lightly.

Furious, my father continued to insist that he was fine, that it was just a blip. But in the end he acquiesced.

It took longer to convey the message that he should gradually withdraw from the office and start by taking rest days at home.

'It makes sense, Dad,' I said. 'That way you can conserve your energy.'

By mid-July he had taken this advice and did, occasionally, spend a day at home. But on these days he fretted terribly, and drove me and his other colleagues mad with his confused and anxious phone calls. He couldn't let go and kept checking if various tasks had been performed in his absence.

But the days when he did insist on going into the office, badgering my mother to drive him in, were even worse – for all of us. His days were in no way productive, but we played along. The staff, my mother, myself and all his senior colleagues were complicit in the charade in which he felt he was doing genuine work.

Working together, we created small phantom tasks for him. And we rang his friends and former colleagues asking them to visit for 'meetings'. Tired of the fruitless arguments, we now told him whatever he wanted to hear, whatever calmed him down – abandoning any semblance of the true state of affairs.

His state of denial could not go on. And it didn't. On Wednesday 31 July 1985, he went with my mother to see a neurologist to get the results of some cognitive tests. My mother had discussed this appointment with me, ringing frequently to list her fears and anxieties. I was busy at work in the TEAM office that day and asked her to report the findings to me. She rang in the middle of the afternoon. Answering, all I could hear were deep, heart-rending sobs. And though, whatever the outcome, I expected her to be upset, I was taken aback by the note of anger in her voice – that, along with despair.

'He was so rude,' she wailed. 'So dismissive.'

'Who?' Was she talking about the doctor or my father?

'The neurologist, of course! He was so impatient.'

'But what did he say? What's wrong?'

'He rattled it off. He said your father has to quit his work immediately.'

'I see! I don't suppose he took *that* one well.'

She harrumphed. 'You know your father.' There was a pause, and then, her voice rising with indignation she said, 'And he said *I* must quit work too.'

'Oh.' I hadn't expected that, and knew it must have come as a body blow. Although her career was waning, my mother was still picking up a few character roles. The previous year she had appeared as Mrs Callaghan in the TV series *The Irish R.M.*

'Why?' I asked, tentatively.

'I have to be at home to mind him.'

'I'm so sorry. But is there a diagnosis?'

'Well, he said it's advanced dementia, but your father's not having it.' She blew her nose loudly. 'That awful insufferable man just told us those facts, bluntly. Advanced dementia, and he needs full-time care at home.' She paused for dramatic effect. 'From me!'

'What else did he say?'

'Nothing! Oh God,' she wailed. 'What are we going to do?'

She didn't put the phone down, and as I offered some unhelpful platitudes I could hear my father in the background. 'The man's a fool,' he muttered. 'There is nothing wrong with me. Nothing at all!'

'Look, Mum,' I said. 'Stay where you are. I'll leave the office now and be with you as soon as I can.'

I gathered my things together and told my colleagues I had to go. I didn't explain the situation. I don't like to bring outside trouble and stresses into work; I try to keep the two things entirely separate.

Cycling to my childhood home, my mother's sobs still ringing in my ears, I knew this event was a real marker. Things were going to change. With a sinking heart I realised our roles had reversed. The child was now the father of the man.

All I could really offer on this last day of July 1985 was my presence and concern, and not much else. I knew in my heart that the diagnosis was undoubtedly correct, and that we had now entered a whole new phase in this traumatic passage. As it happened I had planned, arranged and booked a weekend trip with friends to Leenane in Connemara for the following day. And although my first instinct had been to cancel, and to stick around and help however I could, I reconsidered.

'You need a couple of days to recover,' I said. 'We can regroup on Monday and take things carefully from there.'

Everything had changed and yet, from my father's perspective, nothing had. He continued his policy of denial, continued struggling into work. And this went on until October, when he developed severe pain and ended up in hospital for gall bladder surgery. My mother expressed relief on handing over his care, but the experience did not suit my father. Disorientated and in pain, he became angry and distressed.

Visiting him one evening, I found his bed empty. I panicked and rushed up to the nurses' station, but they pointed down the corridor and there he was, determinedly pacing, papers tucked under his arm, muttering about the meeting he had to attend. I touched his shoulder and said, 'Hello, Dad,' but he shook me off. 'I'll be late,' he said. I tried to talk him down, but his eyes were restless. 'Poor Brennie,' he muttered. This phrase, once uttered in jest, was becoming a catchphrase as his illness progressed.

'It's impossible to have a conversation with him,' said my mother, when I reported back to her. 'How will I cope when he's discharged?'

'He'll be better once he gets home,' I said.

But he wasn't. If anything, his anger increased along with his confusion. It was a vicious circle. The worsening of his symptoms angered him, the anger increased his symptoms, and so it went on. Yet he still fervently believed he was capable of work, even though his career was well and truly over. This was clear to everyone – everyone except him.

The worse my father became, the more my mother depended on me for both practical and emotional support. And the more she depended on me, the more burdened I felt. Then when my brother Julian told me that he had received a posting to New York with Córas Tráchtála, and that he and his family would be moving there soon, I found it difficult to be happy for him.

How could I be, when this meant I would shoulder the burden of our parents alone? I was twenty-eight years old. A young man with ambition. I should be enjoying myself, throwing myself into acting and producing without a care in the world. Full of self-pity, I found myself muttering 'poor Ron-ie', deliberately and ironically adapting my father's mutterings of 'Poor Brennie'.

As well as feeling sorry for myself – and by God I did – I was sinking lower and lower emotionally. I hated seeing him like this! My father, of whom I had been so very proud, even after I had become increasingly aware of the dysfunction, and of his work obsession.

My father was in and out of hospital. I visited, both wanting to and not wanting to. Sometimes I'd find him peaceful and accepting, but more often I'd find him agitated, frustrated and confused.

After one visit when my father, taking my hand, had begged me not to leave him, I sat alone on Patrick Kavanagh's bench on the canal near Baggot Street as darkness fell. Surrounded by discarded fast-food litter, and dwelling on this whole sorry mess, I was appalled to find myself sobbing hysterically. I couldn't stop. Terrified of being seen like this out in public I stood up, took a few deep breaths and, marching furiously along the canal bank, I channelled my upset into red-hot anger. Why did this have to happen to my father? Why was he to be punished? It felt utterly random.

One evening when I arrived at the hospital, he seemed surprised to see me. 'I didn't know you were coming to Paris,' he said. Then, pulling me towards him, he muttered into my ear. 'They're not letting me out of the hotel, Ronan,' he said, pointing at a nurse who was filling in a chart on the other side of the ward. 'Will you please tell them how important my meetings are?' His eyes were wild, his speech rapid and rambling. It was hard to talk him down, and almost impossible to leave him there.

I dreaded visiting the following evening, but to my relief he was sitting in a chair, calm and relaxed. It was, of course, a drug-induced calm, but I was pleased that the doctors had been able to prescribe this stability for him.

My mother rarely visited. 'I hate hospitals,' she'd say when I offered her a lift. 'You know that.'

I called in on her regularly to report on his condition, and she'd say, 'At least he's safe. That's such a blessing.'

If only my father could forget about his world of work. But he couldn't. I sympathised; the theatre had been his life. But he was lucky. His friends and former colleagues, aware of all his many achievements, were still acting to protect him. Nobody wanted his reputation besmirched in any way. Everyone wanted the best for him. I assured him of this fact constantly, but he refused to be comforted.

'I'm needed,' he'd insist, and his distress and panic levels would spiral.

On 10 December 1985, my mother agreed to visit him. He'd had a gall bladder operation earlier in the day, and I barely recognised the small, grey, crumpled man in the hospital bed. My mother, equally shocked, sat beside him and tried to take his hand, but he fought her off and tried to tear the tubes out of his arm and his nose.

'My God, he's a fighter,' said a nurse, admiration in her voice as she struggled to contain him. 'That amount of anaesthetic would have most people knocked out for hours more.' Leaning close to my father she said, 'Try to sleep.'

The following evening I visited alone. My mother said she found it too upsetting. I found my father in a troubled sleep and was struck again with how very thin and weak he had become.

The doctors had mentioned that they suspected he might have cancer, and looking at him now, a shadow of his former self, I had a thought that shocked me: maybe it would be a blessing; a quick death from cancer would allow him to escape from the lingering decline of Alzheimer's. But when the results came back from the operation they were clear: no cancer was detected.

As I absorbed this news, I realised that in a fundamental way I had already begun to pass through the grief of his death. The echo of that old and cruel description of Alzheimer's disease as 'the living death' came back to me.

While I was juggling all my father's concerns, getting increasingly stressed about it all, I continued to hold down my full-time job as Artistic Director of TEAM Theatre. It was hard after a long day having to fit in work for my father each evening, and then to visit him and check on my mother as well. To say that this was a difficult, stressful and exhausting time is to understate it.

For all that, it was a happy time professionally. I loved the challenge of working with writers I admired – playwrights like Frank McGuinness, Bernard Farrell, Neil Donnelly, Jim Nolan and Antoine Ó Flatharta. And I relished my role, believing it to be a good fit for me. I understood the business of theatre and, being an actor, was able to empathise with and relate well to those we employed.

We'd arrive into schools in one van with a very small set and sound system and would set up in a room. It was a small operation, but really magical, especially if you could engage the students, and mostly we could. They were enthusiastic, and we went away thinking, well sure, that was a good day's work. That contrasted with some of the acting jobs I'd taken on in mainstream theatre. Those, mostly small roles, were frankly a bit dull.

One of my roles was to promote theatre education. I was trying to create the beginnings of other companies, and travelled to Cork to visit Graffiti Theatre. I sat in the audience watching its performance of *Othello*, which had been chosen to bring to life the text which was on the Leaving Certificate syllabus. An actress called Miriam Brady was playing Emilia, wife of the villain, Iago.

I saw her later, sitting with the rest of the cast across the staff room from where I was talking to the show's director. I noticed in passing that she was attractive, with a mane of dark hair. I wasn't introduced to her or to any of the cast. I remember feeling that that was a little odd, as their perspective on the work might well have been useful to me, but I didn't ask to talk to them. The purpose of this trip had been to develop a relationship with the director.

A year later we were recruiting new actors for the coming season. Somebody mentioned the name Miriam Brady, and I said, 'Why do I know that name?'

'She was in Graffiti Theatre, down in Cork,' said the producer.

'Ah yes,' I said as it came to me. 'She was in *Othello*, wasn't she?'

'That's right. She played Emilia.'

'Yes.' I shut my eyes, trying to conjure up her face. 'Yes. She was good. Let's give her a try.'

I'm going to let Miriam herself describe our meeting and its aftermath, so the next chapter is hers.

Seven

Miriam's Story

When a producer from the theatre company TEAM rang me, offering me an audition, I wasn't interested. In 1986, after my work with Graffiti Theatre, I had left Ireland for a year to live in Kenya and work with babies who had malnutrition. When I got back, there was no work available.

I'd moved from Dublin when I was twenty and had left my husband of a year to make a new start in Cork. After returning from Kenya and looking for work, it hadn't crossed my mind to leave Cork. I wasn't happy there exactly – having been brought up in Dublin I found the place parochial – but I was settled. And I had my son Brian to consider. He was eight years old and happy in school. The last thing I wanted to do was uproot him and drag him to Dublin.

But as the producer talked on, describing exactly how the company worked and what my role in it would be, I found myself listening intently. 'We perform a huge variety of plays,' he was saying. 'The first one is by Jim Nolan. It's called *Dear Kenny* and there's a nice part for you. I think you'd fit in well,' he said. 'It's a small company, a bit like a family.'

I liked the sound of that. At twenty-seven I had clocked up a lot of acting experience, but this company, which produced such a variety of roles, would progress my career. I asked for time to think about it and, when I did, I decided that this was an opportunity not to be missed. The producer rang back a week later, and I agreed to travel to Dublin before Christmas for the audition.

There was just one problem, one that left me light-headed with nerves. I remembered TEAM's Artistic Director Ronan Smith, and I was worried about having constant proximity to him. I'd only seen him once and that was over a year earlier. I'd never spoken to him yet he had come into my mind since – and even into my dreams.

I had seen him across the staff room after the performance of *Othello*, and there was just something about him. He was wearing a tweed jacket, I remember, and stylish brown leather brogues. I don't know why I remember the shoes; I suppose, being highly polished and well cared for, they contributed to the impression that here was a gentleman. Surreptitiously watching him as he chatted to our producer, something changed in me; I had this strange stomach-clenching reaction.

I turned to my friend Colette and said, 'I'm going to marry that man.'

She stared over at him. 'He looks nice,' she said.

'He's a Mr Darcy.'

Colette laughed. 'And we all know how much you love Jane Austen.'

I told myself not to be so stupid. After all I was going out with someone else, and why would someone so established in the theatre give me a second glance?

I passed my audition and took up my role. I tried very hard to act normally when Ronan Smith was around, but that wasn't easy when even the sight of him could turn me into a quivering wreck. Watching him, I loved his easy manner, and the way he interacted with all the actors. It was obvious from the very first day that everyone in the company loved Ronan. They spoke so warmly of him.

He was steady, he was kind, he was fair and he was very, very funny. He was just great craic. What's more, he had good respect for the actors. And although I retained that fantasy of marrying him, I knew that nothing could possibly happen between us – he wasn't interested. Yet I ached to be close to him. And that heartache got worse and worse as the months went on.

At the end of the year, when schools had broken up for summer, Ronan called me into his office. Running my fingers through my hair, I felt as nervous as if I was going to collect my Leaving Certificate results. This was the day that would determine my future, for the next season at least. All six of us actors had an appointment with him. It was either 'Thank you very much, and goodbye' or 'Would you like to come back next year?' I fervently hoped it would be the latter.

Seeing me, Ronan looked up and smiled. 'Ah, Miriam! There you are.' He shuffled some papers on his desk. 'Miriam, we've really liked the work you've done this year,' he said. 'You've fitted into the company exceptionally well, on and off the stage, and we'd like to offer you work for next year. How does that sound to you?'

I let the silence grow, and was delighted to see that Ronan looked a little anxious. Or was that my imagination working overtime?

'Thank you,' I said. 'I'll think about it.'

'Good! Good!' He smiled. 'Let me know when you've decided.'

I had, of course, already made up my mind to stay with TEAM, but I didn't want to show Ronan just how keen I was.

I couldn't stop smiling as I made my way back to my apartment in Rathgar. I felt like dancing. And that wasn't just because of this new offer of work. It meant another year of being close to Ronan. Maybe something would happen between us. But if I thought that the job offer meant he was interested in me, I realised I was being ridiculous. Word had it that Ronan was in a relationship and, although all of us in the company were good friends and had enjoyed evenings out as a group, he had never shown interest in any of us.

Before I knew it, the long summer break almost over, Ronan rang me.

'Could you pop into the office sometime, please?' he said. 'I've got your script for you here.'

'Do you have a cold?' I asked him. His nasal tones suggested that he had.

'I'm just a bit stuffed up.'

I suspected that Ronan had sinusitis and, being interested in alternative therapies, I went to a health shop and bought a remedy for sinusitis to give him. This was my big gesture. It was a sign saying, 'I care about you.' Would Ronan pick up the signal?

I called into the office the following day, pushed the remedy across the desk and said, 'This is for you.'

Ronan was delighted. 'That's really thoughtful,' he said, thanking me. As he handed me my script across the desk – I was to play a character called Lady Vanessa in a play called *Two Houses* by John McArdle – he glanced up at me. And then, as I turned to go he said very casually, and in a blasé manner, 'I have two tickets for *Summer* by Hugh Leonard. I don't know if you'd like to go?'

I tried not to get excited. 'With you, you mean?'

'Well, yes! It's for the opening night?' Did he think I needed to be persuaded?

I smiled. 'I'd love that.' I paused. 'But there is just one thing. I'll have to get a sitter for Brian.' Did I imagine it or did his face fall? 'But I'm sure I can organise that. What night is it?'

'Wednesday,' he said, as I opened the door and made my way through it. I walked away, wondering to myself was this a date? No! It couldn't be. Ronan saw me as a friend, and I happened to be there. But oh, just suppose that it was!

I felt ridiculously nervous as I waited for him to pick me up, more like a teenager than a divorced mother of twenty-seven years of age. I chose my clothes carefully. I wore a long black fitted skirt that swished at the bottom, teamed with a beautiful Japanese lace blouse given to me by a Japanese friend. I hadn't many clothes, but this, I felt, was perfect for a first night.

The doorbell rang bang on time, and there was Ronan. Smart as ever, he wore navy chino-type trousers, a lovely navy jumper with red bits on the collar, with a collarless shirt underneath and the now-familiar brown brogues. Ever the gentleman, he walked down the steps before me, opened the passenger door of his yellow Citroën Dyane, waited for me to get in and closed it before walking round to the driver's side. When our eyes met I felt a frisson pass between us.

We drove to the theatre in complete silence, apart from the tick tock of the car clock. It wasn't an uncomfortable silence so much as one of anticipation. Was this the start of something? Did Ronan want it to be?

Arriving, we were swept into the Abbey Theatre, which was full of luvvies and prominent personalities from Irish showbusiness. The play, about how the passing of time affects relationships, was highly enjoyable. When we arrived in the bar for a drink after the play, Ronan was hailed by playwrights Tom Murphy and Bernard Farrell. Jane Brennan was amongst the group too. I knew her to say 'Hi' to, because she lived across the road from me in Brighton Square. She had worked with Ronan and welcomed me to the group with a friendly generosity.

I didn't feel out of place, because I was with Ronan, but I didn't contribute much to the conversation. I was acutely aware that I was just a young actor and not part of the Dublin theatre scene. I was extremely shy, and was happy listening to the others. Yet all I really wanted was to be alone with Ronan; all I really wanted was to kiss him.

There was a woman at the end of the bar with dyed strawberry-blonde hair who was being hailed by everyone. She was talking, or rather booming, in an exaggerated, actressy manner. I saw her turn around and make her way towards our group. 'Darling,' she said, throwing her arms around Ronan, 'there you are!' Seeing her proprietorial attitude towards him I realised that this was his mother, the famous Beryl Fagan.

Ronan introduced her to me and she shook my hand. Was she weighing me up, I wondered? Was she comparing me to Ronan's previous girlfriends? Or was I to her just a girl in the company? That was the way that Ronan had introduced me, after all. I couldn't tell, but she didn't seem particularly interested in me. She made vague attempts to include me in the conversation, but I shrank back thinking, 'Oh God – I don't know what to say.' Thankfully, she didn't give me an inquisition.

Ronan finished his pint and refused a second one. He turned to me. 'Shall we leave?' he asked.

'Yes!' I said, with delight. We would be alone again! Back in his car, we chatted easily. We discussed the play, we talked of Brian and of my role as a single mum. When we drew up at my apartment, Ronan left the engine running, but I didn't want him to go. I invited him in for a cup of tea.

He hesitated. Then he said, 'Yes. That would be lovely!'

'Is chamomile okay?' I asked when we entered the kitchen. 'Or would you prefer builder's?'

He chose chamomile so I made it, then joined Ronan on a beanbag; pleased, for once, that my apartment contained so little furniture. Sitting there with my Mr Darcy – looking out through the bay window at the most stunning full moon – I thought it must be the most romantic moment of my entire life. And when Ronan turned towards me and kissed me, it felt like the most natural thing in the world. I felt a bubble of happiness.

But then he pulled away. 'I'm sorry,' he said. 'I'm a bit radioactive at the moment.'

'You're radioactive?'

'What I mean is, my head is all over the place right now. I'm just out of a relationship.'

'I understand,' I said, but he'd burst my bubble.

He kissed me, briefly, on the lips, then said, 'I'd better go home. It's late, and we've work in the morning.'

He didn't ask me out again. Not immediately. But a couple of weeks later I organised a dinner party for all the people who were leaving the company. I cooked a vegetarian meal – I was at it all day – and having Ronan there, along with everyone else, made me uneasy with nerves. Were my feelings for him obvious?

After dinner we all moved on to a nightclub on Leeson Street called Suesey Street. Ronan asked me to dance; I accepted, and he swung me onto the floor. We did the jive and he was such an expert, if vigorous, dancer, that it was easy to fall into his rhythm. He made me feel as if I was equally adept and I loved that sensation, as we continued to dance the night away.

I was on an adrenaline high when finally we walked outside with Jane, the Production Manager. We chatted for a minute or two, then, perhaps sensing that we wanted to be alone Jane waved, walked to her car and drove off.

'We'd better get going too,' said Ronan, rattling his car keys. 'It's getting late.'

I looked at him and shook my head. 'I don't want to go home,' I said. 'Not yet. I don't want the night to end.'

He smiled. 'So,' he said. 'What *do* you want to do? There's not much open at this time of night.'

'Let's go for a lovely walk somewhere,' I said. 'It's such a glorious night.'

'Okay. I'll take you to my very favourite place,' he said, opening the car door and helping me in. He drove to the Pigeon House overlooking Sandymount Strand, and we walked the length of the pier. We watched the lights across the bay and, holding hands, gazed up at the starlit sky.

'It's beautiful,' I said.

He nodded. 'This is where I do all my thinking.'

He was silent for a while, and I wondered what was going through his mind. Then a breeze blew in from the sea and, shivering, I wrapped my arms around myself.

'You're cold,' said Ronan. 'Let me give you my jacket.'

I'd noticed the coat before. It was distinctive. Classic black leather, and it felt heavy as he placed it around my shoulders.

'This is beautiful,' I said, pulling it closer.

'It belonged to my dad. He wore it for years and years. It was almost a part of him.' Then, looking sad, a slump in his shoulders, he said, 'He's in a nursing home now.'

'Yes,' I said. 'I heard that.' I squeezed his hand. 'I'm so sorry.'

'Yeah. Well. At least he's safe there. At least he's not trying to work.'

He didn't kiss me. Not then, but I didn't mind. That didn't stop me from feeling close to him as we walked, his arm around me. We were silent as we walked back down the pier, but it was a comfortable silence. As we reached his car, the sky was turning red in a glorious dawn. 'Wow!' I said. 'Would you look at that!' Then I glanced at my watch. 'Oh my God,' I said. 'You do realise it's six o'clock in the morning?'

We drove home in silence, and Ronan waited while I turned the key and walked into my apartment. As I undressed, cleaned my teeth and crawled beneath my bedclothes, I felt a calm sense of happiness. I didn't stop to wonder why Ronan hadn't come on to me. I was getting to know him and the more I knew, the more I liked. He was, simply, the perfect gentleman.

I already suspected that he was 'the one'. Could he be sensing the same thing? Was that possible? And that, it being so he wanted to take his time, wanted to avoid putting a foot wrong? Whatever it was, I slept deeply, and woke the next day bathed in happiness.

Shortly afterwards, in August 1988, we were both invited to a double wedding. We knew one of the couples – a girl from TEAM was marrying the Traveller actor Michael Collins, and they'd asked pretty much the whole company along. After dinner we danced together. We danced to Roy Orbison, we danced to hits by Elvis. And then a Ben E. King number came on.

'I love Ben E. King,' I said.

'So do I,' said Ronan.

And as that track, 'Stand by Me', played, Ronan snuggled into me and, as I listened to the words of the first verse, something shifted. I just 'knew'. And when he gazed at me, looking so searchingly into my eyes I could swear he could see my soul, and I realised that he felt it too.

When the music ended and the inevitable hangers-on, the worse for drink, started up a raucous sing-song, we took that as our cue to go.

'Come to my place,' said Linda, a friend from the company. 'My apartment is just around the corner.'

When we arrived there we sat on the couch holding hands. Linda made us all tea, we drank it and some while later, wanting to be alone, we left. Ronan drove me home. And from that time on we were a couple.

It was wonderful at first: spending my spare time with Ronan, getting closer and more intimate. But the weight of the relationship began to impinge, and I realised I needed time and space to breathe.

Ronan was a passionate and committed cyclist, and I asked him if I could borrow his bicycle. He agreed, and I took the bike to Connemara, and spent three days cycling around the coast. It was liberating and gave me necessary thinking time. By the time I was due to go home, I was sure that my feelings were real. I couldn't wait to see Ronan again.

We'd decided, before I left, that we'd meet the evening of my return. I planned to go home first to shower and change, but on impulse I cycled straight to Ronan's apartment in Holles Row. Opening the door, he pulled me into a hug.

'I'm cooking for you,' he said, proudly.

I was really touched. He'd gone to a lot of effort and had made lasagne. It wasn't a culinary triumph – the taste of blue cheese dominated the dish – but it was a thoughtful gesture, and one I truly appreciated.

The relationship deepened. We spent any time we could in each other's company. But then Ronan took TEAM on tour to France. I couldn't go because I'd taken on another role, and I missed him terribly.

He rang, telling me that he missed me too. 'Let's get away somewhere when I get home,' he suggested. 'We can spend the weekend miles from anywhere.' He suggested we rent a tiny cottage in Co. Monaghan that some of the company had stayed in when we had toured TEAM to Monaghan and Cavan. I duly booked it.

We arrived in pouring rain and hauled our cases inside. We decided to go for a walk despite the weather, and with the wind whipping my hair across my face, we set off.

It got so bad that we took shelter under a hawthorn tree, our arms around each other for warmth. And in that moment, as we laughed easily together, it struck me forcibly that Ronan was the man for me. Looking into his eyes I thought, 'I want to marry you, maybe I'll ask you,' but at that very moment my hat blew off and travelled with the speed of a frisbee. Releasing me, Ronan ran hell for leather and retrieved it for me. The mood was broken.

We stayed in for dinner. Ronan had bought a special bottle of red wine in France; it was so good that we finished it with the main course and, noticing that, Ronan looked a little disgruntled. I couldn't work out why. But when I tried to snuggle up to him as we sat in front of a smoking peat fire, he held his body rigid.

'Are you okay?' I asked him.

He didn't answer. Instead, he slid himself off the sofa and went down on one knee. I was astonished. 'Miriam, I would really like to spend the rest of my life with you,' he said.

'What on earth do you mean?' I said, in a tone Ronan now describes as my Margaret Thatcher voice. I truly was confused by his choice of words.

Looking a little downcast, he repeated the sentence. 'I would really like to spend the rest of my life with you.'

I stared at him. What, exactly, was he asking me? Was he talking marriage, or did he want us to get, casually, together? And what of Brian? Had he taken my son into account? Would he marry the two of us? Or did he want us all to live in sin for the rest of our lives?

'Well?' He stared up at me with pleading, puppy-dog eyes.

Crossing my arms, I gazed down at him. 'Would you mind if I gave that a bit of thought?'

He shrugged and pulled himself back onto the couch. 'Fair enough,' he said.

We headed for bed soon afterwards, and as we lay together thoughts were looping around my mind. I turned over, hugged him tightly from behind. He relaxed into the hug. 'I can feel your heart beating,' he said, and yawned deeply.

Pushing myself up onto my elbow, I leant over him. 'Ronan.'

'Mmm.'

I took a deep breath and said, loudly and very deliberately, 'Yes.'

'That's great,' he said. And I waited for him to turn over and sweep me into his arms. And I waited. But a minute later he started snoring.

So there I was on the most exciting night of my life. I've decided to live with the love of my life forever, whether or not he has marriage on his mind, and there is absolutely no one to share the news with. There's no champagne. No dancing around the floor. I felt so frustrated. I tried to shake Ronan awake. I was quite rough with him, but he just turned over and muttered that he was exhausted.

When, the following day, we talked it all through, Ronan told me that he had missed me so much in France that work had lost its lustre. 'That's when I decided you were the one for me,' he said. 'When I bought the wine, I promised myself that I would have asked you before the bottle was empty.'

'So that's why you were so tense,' I said, the truth dawning.

'That, and asking you at all,' he said. Then he explained that he had chosen his words carefully. 'I want to marry you, Miriam. Of course I do, but I knew that if I mentioned the word marriage, you'd say, "What the fuck do you mean? I'm already married."'

He had a point. When I'd walked out on my husband we'd been granted an annulment by the church, but not by the state. It was something that needed sorting. Having made the big decision, we decided to marry in a church as soon as we could get all the arrangements made; the state wedding could wait.

Eight

One Chapter Closes

I had assumed that my father's weakness following his operation in 1985 would persuade him that the time had come for him to retire. I was wrong. He insisted on going back to work. It was impossible to stop him.

'I don't know what to do,' said my mother, ringing as his convalescence was starting. 'Can't you simply refuse to drive him in?'

'I've tried that,' she said. 'And he says in that case he'll ring you. When I explain that you're busy enough chasing several jobs, he simply calls a taxi. It's hopeless.'

It was indeed hopeless. And it was all I needed. On the days he got himself to the office, I'd rush there in order to supervise his every action. It was now an exhausting, all-consuming preoccupation.

I ran up and down the stairs in a constant battle to prevent disaster: downstairs to his office where I would tidy and file papers, or make a pretence of it so that I could eavesdrop on his conversations; upstairs to ring the person he had been calling back, to tell them that my father was confused and that they should take no action based on what he'd said. I'd then explain to them what, in reality, needed to be done.

This caused me stress and distress in equal measure. My disloyalty felt like a betrayal. I loved my father and so admired him for his many achievements in theatre, and I wasn't the only one to feel this way. But if his reputation were to remain intact, it was essential that I maintain this conspiracy with his peers.

Essentially, I had to rescue my father from himself in order to help my mother, who had entrusted me with his care.

'We have to keep your father's condition away from the public gaze,' she said.

And if my father was difficult in the office, he was worse at home. The clashes caused by his demanding independence were taking a toll on my mother. A cycle developed where the two of them would row, she would become distressed, and the rows would worsen.

'He's so stubborn,' she'd say, close to tears. 'And he gets himself worked up into the most appalling state. I just can't cope with him anymore.'

When I tackled him, he'd insist that he simply *had* to work. 'I can't trust anyone to handle things right,' he said.

'But you've built up a magnificent team.'

He'd harrumph, and mutter that they were a bunch of fools. 'And I'm perfectly capable of managing things myself,' he'd insist. 'There's *nothing* wrong with me.' He was a cornered animal, desperate and exhausted, but bloody-minded and determined too. Something would have to be done. We enlisted the help of his GP.

He listened to all that we had to say, and then said, 'Well I'm sorry, but there's only one thing for it. If he won't rest, if he insists he has to work, then it's time to get him into twenty-four-hour care.'

He booked my father into St John of God Hospital in the south of the city, and my mother, saying she was unequal to the task of driving him in, insisted that I should do this. I assumed she'd accompany the two of us, but when I arrived at their house my mother handed me his packed suitcase and said, 'I'm sorry Ronan. I just can't face it.'

My father appeared, his briefcase bursting with a tangle of papers. I helped him strap into the car.

'This is nonsense,' he said, as I drove.

'I'm sorry?'

'All these visits to doctors and hospitals. It's ridiculous!'

'They're trying to help, Dad,' I said. 'And if you let them, they will.'

'But they don't!' He was restless, his eyes staring around. 'They waste time with all these appointments that go nowhere, and I'm sick of it. Sick of it! I need to be at work.' So saying, he took random papers out of his brief-case, looked at them, not really reading them, and shuffled them around mindlessly before stuffing them back in again.

He continued to vent, and I let him. There was no point doing anything else, since he was hardly likely to cooperate. So I humoured him as best I could until we reached St John of God's car park. And then I lied to him.

'Here we are,' I said, opening the boot to retrieve his case before helping him out of the car. 'Just another day's observation in the hospital.'

When, after various form-filling, he was admitted, we'd located his bed, and I'd unpacked his clothes and toiletries – placing them in the locker – I lied to him a second time. 'Don't worry about a thing,' I said. 'I'll be back to pick you up later, and I've taken all the notes for work – look!' I held out a sheaf of paper with fabricated notes, ready to stick in a bin on my way out. Sitting on a chair, he seemed mollified.

Then a nurse, beckoning me, muttered that I must leave quickly. 'He'll be fine,' she said. 'He'll soon settle, but just leave. And don't look back.'

I tried to follow her instructions – I really did – but as I reached the door, I felt compelled to turn and check on him. And I saw on his face the deep hurt of a lost child. Turning, I shut my eyes briefly, trying to banish the sight from my mind. But it was useless. The incontrovertible truth was this: I was abandoning my father. Disowning him.

Walking swiftly away from the hospital, away from my problems and responsibilities, I felt like Judas. His face in that moment still haunts me today.

I had thought that, with my father safe and removed from events, my life might become somewhat easier. But my workload increased. My father had left the Olympia Theatre's finances in a precarious state. I worked hard to turn this situation around and ensure that the theatre was in the best of health. It was the least I could do to preserve his legacy.

It was vital to hold the ship steady and to prevent the business from going under. If it collapsed too soon after my father's involvement, blame could be laid at his door, thus ending all his years of struggle on a sour note.

And holding the Olympia together really *had* been a struggle. In 1974, when the proscenium arch (the frame surrounding the stage space) fell, necessitating a costly restoration, this was seen by many as a death knell for the theatre. It had been a huge struggle to turn events around, and the reopening of the theatre after a long and substantial campaign to raise the finance, was seen as a remarkable achievement. Although many people had helped to achieve this, my father's role had been pivotal. The theatre was important to him, and he had driven the agenda with a fierce insistence, day and night.

The Olympia needed new blood. Retaining my role as Company Secretary, I contacted various prominent theatre producers and promoters, offering them directorship roles in the Olympia. I was delighted when I'd achieved this, but I hadn't reckoned on the new directors' egos. Each of them was convinced that their way was the only way – and it was my job to keep the harmony.

Containing these confrontations and shifting alliances took time and effort, and all this had to happen once I'd finished my day job with TEAM. There was little time for any life outside work. What time there was I spent visiting my father, who moved after a while to Bloomfield Nursing Home, a short walk from my parents' house.

There was one thing to be grateful for. The Dublin Theatre Festival was out of my hands. Michael Colgan had taken over, and it was sailing on effectively. My father's two big flagships were safe, and his achievements in both projects had been preserved. I breathed a deep sigh of relief.

The visits to my father proved increasingly difficult. The very sight of me caused him agitation. And the longer I stayed, the more stressed he became. In turn, seeing him like that caused me deep distress. One evening a nurse took me aside. 'The problem,' she said, 'is that you remind your father of his work. He obsesses about it and worries about all the tasks that need doing.'

I'd feared as much. 'What should I do?'

'This will sound harsh,' she said, 'but maybe you should visit less often?'

I nodded, seeing the sense of this. I left that evening with mixed feelings. There was relief, certainly, because the visits were so draining, but there was also guilt.

Over the coming weeks I struggled to follow the new regime. There were times that I really wanted to visit him – he was my father and I loved him. I'd stop myself for his own good and then, thinking about him sitting there alone, seeing other patients receiving visitors, I'd wish that I *had* visited. But when I did visit, I often regretted that too. It had become a no-win situation.

I sank into a dark place. When life got too much, I'd walk out along the Pigeon House Pier in Ringsend. I'd howl, shouting out all my frustration, wishing the wind could carry my problems out to sea.

My mother had moved by this time. She still lived close to the nursing home, but she visited my father even less than I did, and she never went alone. I dreaded the times I accompanied her, because she simply could not cope. She'd try to get him to talk sensibly, and when he couldn't she'd shout at him. She'd reminisce about the past and challenge him to remember the various events – something he was now quite unable to do. In the end, giving her the same advice that the nurse had given me, I discouraged her visits.

Over time, as the disease progressed, it mastered him more and more completely. In one way this was a relief, both for him and for me. He became benign and calm in himself. Instead of constantly fretting he was content to sit still and make small talk. Very small talk. Neither of us mentioned the word 'work', and he rarely asked about my mother. He began to surrender to the illness until he came to be a smiling, very gentle presence. It was strangely peaceful.

My relief was tinged with profound grief, but I felt able to hide that from him. Not so my mother. On her increasingly rare visits, she was still unable to let him be. When she talked to him she'd demand answers, and even at this stage became upset and angry at his failure to respond.

'It's torture seeing him like that,' she'd say as we left. And she would scrabble for a tissue as her tears started to fall.

Much as I wished my mother would be better around my father, I did understand how difficult it all was for her. My mother had always been mentally delicate – or to put it less kindly, rather neurotic – so she took her husband's deterioration very much to heart. She loved him still, of that I am certain, and she was hurt by the illness. She would take it personally, berating God and the angels. 'Where's God when he's needed?' she'd mutter. Then, looking up as if towards heaven she'd shout, 'What the fuck are you doing to this man?'

Visiting in December 1988, I found my father slumped in a wheelchair. I did a double take, appalled to realise that this thin, sunken and frail man, his head drooping, was indeed my father. He couldn't speak. And for the first time, shockingly, he didn't know who I was. This wasn't living! He was in a completely alternate reality. I wanted this to end for him. I wanted it to end now.

On my next visit, as I talked to him – of anything and nothing – he whispered something in return. Leaning towards him, putting my ear close to his mouth I asked him to repeat it.

'Pardon,' he said.

As I repeated the nonsense I'd been uttering, I thought of the appropriateness of that word. Because I did, of course, pardon him. I pardoned him for his obsessive working habits and his absence from the family when we were growing up. I squeezed his hand in acknowledgment and turned from him to hide my tears.

By this time, I had been working as Artistic Director in TEAM for five years. The role had been every bit as fulfilling as I had imagined it might be when the offer first came – I was well suited for the work and was pleased with all that I had achieved. It had ticked all the boxes, but now I felt that new hands were needed to ensure that the mission and vision of the company remained fresh. It was time for me to return to an acting career.

So resolved, I met with John Coolahan, the Chairman of TEAM at the time. John was a very eminent academic in the Irish education sector who worked with various institutions, and took all his many duties extremely seriously. Not wanting to leave the company in the lurch, I intended to see the 1989 season out, so I gave him ample notice to allow for a successor to be found and for careful planning to be carried out.

I hadn't expected Coolahan to be delighted with my news, but even so his reaction surprised me. 'I have to say Ronan, I'm surprised,' he said, looking at me over his half-moon spectacles. 'I thought you'd been happy with TEAM. And we're more than happy with you.'

I told him my reasons and he sat back, regarding me steadily. 'Are you sure, Ronan?'

I assured him that I was.

'Yes, but have you *really* thought this through?'

I nodded, but he said, 'Ronan, take a little time to think about this, will you? Jobs like this don't grow on trees, and it seems to me the role suited your abilities particularly well. Come back to me in a week or two.'

I promised that I would, but during those weeks an event happened which deepened my resolve. My father's birthday was on 7 February. He was turning seventy-two, and I duly paid him a visit. But when I arrived at the nursing home the doctor was waiting to talk to me.

'I'm sorry to be the bearer of bad news,' he said. 'Your father has had a series of seizures, or epileptic fits.'

'Epileptic fits?' I was horrified.

'It's not uncommon in Alzheimer's patients,' he said. 'But I have to warn you, his condition could herald a crisis.'

'You mean he could have more fits?'

He shrugged. 'We really don't know what exactly this might mean – but there could be a drastic change sooner rather than later.'

I let his words sink in, then nodded. I understood what was being signalled, but not explicitly said. My father could die at any time.

This was foremost in my thoughts when I met with John Coolahan again.

'I haven't changed my mind,' I said. 'I'm sure I've made the right decision, both for me and for the good of TEAM.'

'Oh.' He didn't look happy. 'You're going to resign?'

'Yes,' I said. 'I'm sorry, but I am. But I won't let you down. I'll see out the season, as I promised.'

John looked at me meditatively as I left his office, gently closing the door behind me. I *was* sure that it was the right decision – that it was time for a change – but that didn't stop me from being grateful for his obvious and sincere concern.

Knowing that he truly had my best interests at heart had made me realise, in a stark moment, how much I was missing my father's concern and advice. Over the next months I paid more frequent, but ever-briefer visits. There was little to say and while I hoped my presence was a comfort, I had no way of knowing if he even knew I was there. Although still physically present, he was now entirely absent.

My mother shared John Coolahan's fears for me, and told me forcefully that I was mad to give up a steady job to return to the desperate uncertainty of freelance acting, but much of her opposition stemmed from her fear of how my change of direction would affect *her*.

'You'll be away a lot, touring,' she said when I went to tell her the news. 'And it's not the best time with your father the way he is.' There was real fear in her eyes.

I wasn't leaving TEAM entirely empty-handed. I had met and fallen in love with the actress Miriam Brady, who had joined the company of TEAM during my term there. We had become close over the past year and were now spending a great deal of time together. She had proved a wonderful support and a listening ear over the past difficult months.

The last, even more difficult months as I worked out my notice, staying until the end of the season as I'd promised, saw my stress levels soar exponentially.

It was in early March 1989 that I was invited to be a guest on *The Late Late Show* to talk to Gay Byrne about my father's Alzheimer's journey. After this, I began to undertake some advocacy work for better awareness and understanding of dementia.

Work was challenging enough. We were going through the final rehearsals and first previews of TEAM's new play, *The Native Ground*, written for us by Antoine Ó Flatharta. It was a powerful play which examined the tension between Travellers and the settled community, and tried to tease out the basis for fear and antagonism between the groups. I was determined to make this work well, and was pleased with the way the cast of five was shaping up. Miriam was excellent as Eithne, one of the settled members of the cast.

Leaving the rehearsals with adrenaline coursing through my veins, and my stress levels stratospheric, the visits to my father proved to be more than I could bear. And were they worthwhile? It was impossible to know. Observing the empty shell that was my father, utterly incapable of connecting, I'd talk to myself.

'What am I doing here?' I'd say out loud, as I thought of all the work I could have, and indeed, should have been catching up on.

In spite of the doctor's fears, there was little change in my mute father as one month followed another. And my visits became something of a stopped-clock experience, occurring outside time. It was a torturous, alternate reality that existed in a separate dimension.

His death finally came on 31 October 1989. The nursing home rang me with the news, telling me he had slipped away most peacefully. My first call was to Julian, who had recently returned from New York.

He absorbed the news silently. I heard him take a deep breath before asking, 'Does Mum know?'

'Not yet. I thought we could both tell her,' I said. 'It's not news to give over the phone, and I want to prepare her gently.'

Julian suggested that we should tell her over dinner. 'Bring her over to my house this evening,' he said.

I did so. Miriam came too, to give me moral support, and when we arrived she went to say goodnight to my young nieces, leaving Julian and me to deliver the bad news. There was no easy way to do this. We put off the moment, engaging in small talk for a while, and then we told her.

She let out a loud, low groan. A truly shocking sound, like a wounded deer.

'No. No. No.' Putting her hands over her face, she howled, and sobbed, noisily. Then she grabbed for a handful of tissues from the box that I held out to her.

Julian and I exchanged a look of puzzlement. We'd expected her to be sad, but surely his death couldn't have taken her by surprise? Unless she had harboured some strong secret denial, or an irrational hope of a recovery? Could she have? Or was this a form of a necessary rite she was impelled to go through? Being unused to grief myself, I honestly couldn't guess.

Watching her, absorbing her very real, profound distress, I wondered at our differing reactions. My emotions did not resemble hers at all. I had been grieving for years already, acutely missing the man he had been, mourning the loss of his true essence. I saw his death as a welcome release for him and, in all honesty, for me too. Looking at Julian, noticing his surprise at the violence of our mother's reaction, I think he felt the same as I did.

Miriam wasn't surprised. 'I expected that reaction,' she said as we drove home later. 'That's why I went to see Jill,' she added, talking of my three-year-old niece. 'As soon as I heard the screaming, I started singing to Jill to drown your mother out.'

'Singing?'

'Yes – operatically! And the louder the howling became the louder my singing got. I put on quite a performance, I can tell you!'

I laughed. 'What did Jill make of that?'

'Oh, she's used to me fooling around – you know she is. This was just her mad Aunty Miriam.'

My father's funeral, which took place in Donnybrook Church, was a grand affair. President Hillery was abroad at the time, but he sent a representative, and many dignitaries from Irish public life attended along with the expected contingent from the world of theatre and the arts.

I regarded the day as one to simply get through. I'd held on to my anger for all the struggling and suffering my father had made for himself and for those of us around him, but my mother, herself a very public figure, took real comfort from the respect and regard shown for him. What would become of her now? And, more pertinently, what would she expect from me? Would I become her surrogate husband? Time would tell.

This wasn't quite the end of Dad's story. I wanted to remember him, but I also wanted his story to be of use to others. And it was for this end that I continued my work with the ASI for another year, staying on the board and working supportively with the Chairman, Michael Coote.

I admired Michael enormously. Retired from a successful senior management role, he had cared for his wife when she contracted Alzheimer's. Then, using his exceptional skills and energy, he transitioned the ASI from an organisation run by volunteers into a professional and highly effective entity backed by public funds – so allowing the society to deliver services.

There was a little opposition from those members of the board who had acted as founding members, and I became a kind of diplomat, easing the transition and assuring them that the right steps were being taken.

The transition worked well. And when I felt assured that our first professional executive employee had settled in, and that the enlarged board was working well, I felt it was my time to go.

Resigning from the board, wishing them well, I put the whole issue of Alzheimer's behind me. Now it was time to get on with my own life.

Nine

Acting Again

Shortly after my father's death, I gained a part in the Abbey Theatre's production of Seán O'Casey's *The Shadow of a Gunman*, playing the part of an English soldier. For this role I had to perfect a cockney accent. We toured Ireland from November 1989, then came the exciting news that we were to take the play overseas and tour Australia and New Zealand. This was a first for the Abbey Theatre.

We left to great fanfare in March 1990; this was just three months before Miriam and I were set to marry. It was hard saying goodbye to her. I felt bad, knowing that she would now have to cope alone with all our marriage plans. We'd made a start, we had chosen her antique lace wedding dress and picked out a smart, yet bohemian outfit for me. And we had bought our wedding rings. But there was still a great deal to be done.

Before I left I wrote a series of love letters on postcards to Miriam, placed them in envelopes and asked a friend to post them for me, one for every week that I was away.

The tour was sold out before we'd even left Ireland, so we played to packed houses. After opening on 31 March at the Adelaide Theatre Festival, we moved on to New Zealand to take part in the arts festival in Wellington, before returning to Australia and finishing the tour in Perth, Western Australia.

Although the pressures engendered by my father's illness were now behind me, my responsibilities did not cease. His death, if anything, had increased my mother's need for support. She would ring constantly, wanting both help and company. Conscious that the timing of the tour wasn't good for Mum, Miriam had assured me that she would keep an eye on her while I was away.

'There's one thing I'd really love you to do,' I said to Miriam after one of my mother's more 'poor me' phone calls.

'What's that?'

'Could you act as her surrogate husband?'

'Her what?' Miriam spluttered with laughter, then coughed as her tea went down the wrong way.

'Escort her to the theatre now and then. It's one of the things she expects from me. You know how much she loves that.'

She agreed, if rather reluctantly. 'I just hope she behaves herself,' said Miriam. 'Unlike at *The School for Scandal*!'

We laughed. Miriam had accompanied Beryl to the first night of the Abbey Theatre's production of Richard Brinsley Sheridan's play, in which I was acting. The play requires frequent and rather complex scene changes and, being inventive, the Artistic Director, Patrick Mason, wanted to avoid a blackout between scenes, so they had to be stylised.

Instead of using stage management to carry out this furniture-removing role, Patrick had decided to allocate members of the cast to do the job. And I was one of those selected. On the third or fourth scene change, the unmistakable voice of my mother rang out clearly through the theatre. 'Wait until I get Patrick,' she said. 'I'm going to kill him!'

I was alarmed at the time, and snatched a surreptitious glance at Patrick who sat, stony-faced, near the front of the theatre. But afterwards Miriam and I had a good laugh about it.

'I could feel it was coming,' she said. 'Beryl so clearly thought that such menial tasks were unfit for someone of her darling son's status! But the worst thing,' she said, 'was that people clearly thought it was my fault and that I should have been able to shut her up.'

'Poor you,' I said, but I was still laughing.

'Anyway,' I said now, 'with me on the other side of the world, at least you'll be safe from that behaviour.'

Some weeks later, when I rang home from Australia, Miriam told me she was to accompany Beryl to a Russian production of a Chekhov play. The following week, before I'd had a chance to ask her how the evening had gone, Miriam said, 'Your mother is such a snob!'

'What's she done now?'

'Only hummed her way through the whole perfor-mance. Just to show how utterly unimpressed she was.'

'Was it a bad performance?

'That's the thing – no – they were an excellent company!'

Although they got on well enough, Miriam always felt that Beryl didn't accept her. 'I'm not good enough for her darling son,' she said. 'And I can see why.'

'What do you mean?'

'I'm a single parent who has left her husband. I can see why she mightn't like that.'

I returned on 13 May, leaving thirteen days until our wedding on 26 May 1990. Miriam had planned the wed-ding down to the tiniest detail. I arrived with Philip Lee, my best man, at the Blue Church in Kilternan, and waited anxiously for Miriam to appear.

As the string quartet began to play, I turned and saw Miriam framed in the doorway, the sunlight behind her as she walked slowly up the aisle. When she arrived at my side, and smiled, I was stunned by her beauty and grace, and tears of happiness filled my eyes. I took in her antique lace dress and said, 'You look beautiful!'

The music played on. As it drifted to the end, my mother's voice rang out behind me.

'Thank God that's over!'

I raised an eyebrow and we both stifled a giggle. But she couldn't spoil our day. Nobody could.

As the ceremony progressed I fell into a happy trance. Then when we said our vows, and exchanged our antique rings, I found myself choked with emotion at the significance of this life-shaping ritual and the beauty of the love and hope it celebrated.

The weather was kind to us, and we spilled out of the church into glorious sunshine and mingled amongst our guests. Then we left for the reception, which we held in the garden of Castletown House in Kildare. Wanting to surprise Miriam, I played 'Tabhair Dom Do Lámh' on the flute. That means 'Give Me Your Hand'.

I wondered with some nervousness what the content of Philip's speech would be. As my oldest friend, he had a surfeit of material, of stories he could have told from our days sharing a flat, but he surprised me. He claimed that he knew before I did that I would marry Miriam. He said he knew it from one phone call.

'Ronan had mentioned girls to me before,' he said, 'but I knew, from when he told me he had a new girlfriend and started to talk of Miriam, from the way he described her, that this was different. I said to him, "Ronan, you don't know it yet, but you are going to marry that girl."' And looking round at all the guests with a sweep of his arm he said, 'And wasn't I right! I was absolutely sure that this day would come. Will you please all raise your glasses to the happy couple.'

Miriam welled up with emotion as everyone toasted us. 'I didn't know you talked about me, way back then,' she said. 'But I suppose that's your reticence. It's the Mr Darcy in you.'

I laughed. Loving Jane Austen, and especially *Pride and Prejudice*, Miriam always liked to call me her Mr Darcy.

We bought a three-bedroom Edwardian terraced house in the village-like Dublin suburb of Rathmines and, almost as soon as we were settled in, an exciting job opportunity came my way. My colleagues and friends Ben Barnes and Arthur Lappin asked me to join them in Groundwork, the company they had set up in 1988 based at The Gaiety Theatre. I accepted eagerly, as this was a chance to marry the arts of acting and producing.

Then in the autumn, Miriam was offered a part in RTÉ's *Glenroe*. The soap, based in Co. Wicklow, aired every Sunday evening and was something of an institution across Ireland. She played the part of Julie Connors, who was married to Johnny, a Traveller. It was a wonderful opportunity for her. She loved the work and made close friends, but best of all it was regular work – and that is not to be sniffed at in the fickle world of acting.

In the early 1990s, mining the rich seam of plays by John B. Keane, Groundwork put on productions of *The Year of the Hiker* and *Moll*. I played the priest in the latter, sell-out production, which starred Barry McGovern and Mick Lally, and Pat Leavy as Moll, the housekeeper.

When I asked Ben Barnes, the Artistic Director, how I should play the priest he said, 'Do that wimp thing you do so well,' and my heart sank. Would I *never* get away from this typecasting?

The play sold out and generated a great deal of money for the company, and for me and Miriam. This enabled us to go on holiday to Australia in 1993 to visit Miriam's sister in Sydney. By now we'd had the happiest news. Miriam was pregnant with our first child. And when Hannah was born later in the year, I was over the moon. She was a beautiful baby and turned into a delightful toddler.

Our run of good fortune continued with productions of *The Chastitute*, *The Man From Clare*, *Sive* and *The Field*. Most of these were staged in The Gaiety Theatre. I continued to combine my acting roles with production and management work, something that suited me very well.

These were both enjoyable and successful working years, and the approach of marrying high production values with strong casting of prominent actors such as Mick Lally, Brendan Gleeson, Pat Leavy and others delivered large and appreciative audiences. Many of these were a new, young cohort who we were introducing to John B. Keane's entertaining, visceral and insightful plays. So having been originally staged for audiences who experienced a 'This is us' feeling, we were now giving the next generation of audiences an 'Oh, so that was what my parents' world was like' experience.

There was, however, a downside. In throwing myself into work – in acting, managing and producing – I was leaving myself little free time. I suppose, since my father's death, I had relished being able to do this without being torn in two by my commitments to him, but I was married now. Miriam, alone with baby Hannah in Rathmines, saw little of me.

When I was asked to give fencing coaching to the actor Armand Assante, who was starring in a TV production of *Kidnapped*, I accepted eagerly. The cast was filming on location in Luggala in the Wicklow mountains, home to Garech Browne of the Guinness clan. When the director realised I was an actor, he also gave me a small part in the movie.

I joined a band of Irish actors: Brendan Gleeson, Alan Stanford, Don Wycherley, Gerard McSorley and David Kelly. As part of a scarlet-clad army I played a Corporal, and on one particularly glorious morning we marched down the hill, the blue cloudless skies above us in stark contrast to the appropriately Guinness tones of Lough Tay nestled below.

And down to the left where cars were parked, I noticed Miriam standing and holding two-year-old Hannah, who was balanced on the bonnet, a picnic laid out beside them. And this shout came across, 'My Daddy! My Daddy!' Could life have been more perfect!

The two of them visited a few more times. And when filming finished, she and Hannah would, occasionally, visit me at the theatre. 'If I don't, you'll never set eyes on Hannah!' said Miriam, and I knew she was right – another echo of the way things had been in my childhood.

This was a common complaint of Miriam's, but I brushed off her concerns. I was happy at work, and got a buzz from it all by being able to play to my strength. It took an outsider to bring me down to earth. Hearing of my work commitments, a man I'd met casually looked puzzled. 'So you work all your waking hours then?' I nodded, and he said, 'Well, watch yourself. Nobody can keep that up indefinitely.'

I was stunned. His advice was too true, and so, so obvious. The stranger somehow broke through my denial. I *was* missing Hannah's babyhood; what kind of a dad did that make me? The same kind of dad as Brendan had been to me, I realised with a sickening awareness. Like my father, I was showing signs of workaholism, and the reality that had marred my childhood was in danger of marring Hannah's in the same way. Why had I been resisting facing this truth? Was I simply too drunk on the success of events to see the truth in Miriam's wise counsel?

As this dawning awareness began to emerge, even as these realities were beginning to sink in, fate intervened. Buoyed by its success, Groundwork decided to branch out. Determined to take on an ambitious major project for the summer season, we decided to stage an extravagant production of the musical *Guys and Dolls*, to be co-produced by a leading British regional theatre company. It seemed like a no-brainer.

We worked flat out during the busy production and rehearsal period, and were happy when we launched the musical to an enthusiastic first-night crowd. But nothing can be certain in the theatre world, and our projected large audience numbers simply failed to materialise after that first-night flurry.

That particular summer, 1995, turned out to be that rare thing in Ireland: a long, scorching one with sunny, warm evenings in which to luxuriate outdoors. This alone would have made selling theatre tickets a tricky enough prospect, but an even bigger problem arose, namely the first full staging of *Riverdance* in the Point Theatre (now the 3Arena) in Dublin. How could our production hope to go up against the frankly awesome competition of that particular phenomenon?

Riverdance attracted huge global interest, creating an irresistible magnet that hoovered up full houses nightly. We were truly vanquished, and in early summer 1996, Groundwork joined the legions of honourable defeats in the volatile world of commercial theatre. The company had to be wound up, and another chapter in my working life ended suddenly and finally. It was sobering. I was now the father of two – my son Loughlin had been born in February, so there was an extra mouth to feed.

Watching my mood of despondency, Miriam said that this could be a blessing. 'It gives you the opportunity to build a more balanced life,' she said. 'And this time, please Ronan, take that chance. We need you. All three of us do.'

Which was all very well, but as the main breadwinner I needed to work, and acting jobs were thin on the ground.

Shortly afterwards my mother died. When she was first diagnosed with the lung disease fibrosis, after a lifetime of smoking, she was still able to live life well. But the illness caught up with her and, in the end, her death in St Vincent's was quick and fairly sudden. The hospital rang one summer's evening, and I was by her side with Miriam as she took her last breath. Looking out of the window, afterwards we saw the sun setting in reds and golds over Dublin Bay.

When my agent rang to tell me that there were Americans in town casting for an advertisement, I thought I might as well try my luck. 'It's great money,' she said. The audition was to take place in one of those old Georgian buildings that Dublin does so well. To get to the waiting area I had to pass the room where the auditions were taking place. Peeping in, I saw the actor Gerry Walsh through the open door. As I made my way up the next flights of stairs I heard the producer giving Gerry his instructions.

'You have to be a chicken,' he was told.

A chicken? I was auditioning to be a chicken? I stopped dead in my tracks. It didn't matter how good the money was, *that* was the ultimate humiliation. I turned on my heel and exited the building.

I was telling the story to my old friend Philip Lee when we met for lunch later that week. Having spent many years abroad, Philip was now back in Dublin, where he had set up, very successfully, in law practice. He laughed, then said that he had a proposition for me.

This was odd.

'How would you like to work with me? You'd be a great asset to the company.'

'Go back to law, you mean?' I was gobsmacked.

'Why not? You'd make a brilliant lawyer,' he said. 'I always said so. You've got a far sharper and more legalistic brain than I do.'

He went on to point out the benefits of a steady nine-to-five office job with a regular pay cheque. 'Your life would be a lot less stressful,' he said.

I was flattered by his offer and felt I shouldn't dismiss it out of hand. Philip had uncanny insight, and his level-headed advice had always been valuable to me. And he was often right. Wasn't he the first one to predict my marriage to

Miriam? And he had done so long before I had any inkling that she and I would go the distance.

But now he was asking me to leave the world of theatre, a world I'd been immersed in for my whole life. Wasn't that a step too far? Theatre was all I knew. It was in my blood. Thanking him profusely and telling him I was grateful for his concern, I turned down the offer and continued to look for a job in theatre. And a bizarre and unusual prospect sailed into view right on cue.

Wealthy New York producers wanted to stage *JFK: A Musical Drama* in Dublin as a try-out for what they hoped could be a major Broadway musical. Ireland, they decided, was the obvious place to do so. It was where the Kennedy family had its roots, and where there was a strong loyalty and pride in the family's achievements.

As a local who knew the territory, I was offered the role of Line Producer. This meant I must deliver all that was required for the project – the cast, the musicians, the set builders, the technical crew – in short, everything.

I was delighted to be on board, and threw myself into what turned out to be a rather bizarre project. Regarding the enterprise as something of a hobby, the wealthy backers of the musical were happy to pay out extremely good rates. Everyone was happy! And, as Miriam said at the time, luck was on my side, as it had been so often throughout my life.

The show opened in the Olympia Theatre on 24 April 1997, with great fanfare. It was due to run for eight weeks. It didn't. Proving to be a bit of a damp squib, it closed after just ten nights. Frank Kilfeather, writing in *The Irish Times* said, 'Can you remember where you were, the night they said JFK has been "shut"!'

This, clearly, was a blow. Aware that the backers had lost a great deal of money, I waited for the flak to fly. But the backers accepted the closure with equanimity. And instead of censuring me, they clapped me on the back and raised their glasses to us all, in thanks.

'We've had a wonderful time in Dublin,' they said, as the wrap party moved into the small hours.

All the Irish that I had hired were happy too. The work might have been briefer than they had hoped, but the money had been good, and fair. They were putting food onto the tables of their families. It was win-win all round.

If the *JFK* project was a piece of luck, then the next venture to present itself was utterly life-changing. The global phenomenon that was *Riverdance* came calling. My future for the next few years was going to be secure.

Ten

Riverdance

Few who saw it could forget that night in 1994 when *Riverdance* unleashed itself upon the world, starting out as a seven-minute interval act during the Eurovision Song Contest. Bringing Irish dance and music bang up to date, the show heralded a newly confident Ireland – one we were happy to identify with and celebrate. It stunned all watchers into an awestruck silence.

When the full-length show stormed to success in the Point Theatre I focused, wryly, on the contrast between *Riverdance* and *Guys and Dolls*. Although *Riverdance* had certainly paved the way to disaster for Groundwork, there was no doubting its reach and appeal. Ireland, and indeed the world, had never seen anything like it.

Since that summer, my friend and colleague Julian Erskine had joined the production, working for Abhann, the company owned by that powerful alliance of Producer Moya Doherty and Director John McColgan.

Riverdance was going global and, as Executive Producer, Julian was in charge of supervising and managing the now multiple productions of the show. At *Riverdance*'s early touring stages, with three productions on the road, the company was fast discovering what a behemoth this production would one day be.

Julian rang me from Germany. 'Ronan,' he said, 'I need your help.' The problem, he said, was that he had to go to America, but that he couldn't in all conscience leave Germany. 'I'm cracking at the seams here,' he said. 'I simply can't be in two places at once.'

'What would you need me to do?'

It turned out there were some personnel problems. People needed to be hired and fired. Would I be interested in joining the company in a new role of Contracts Manager? I smiled at this. Of course I would! Who wouldn't relish the opportunity to jump on board this remarkable global adventure?

Frankly, I was flattered that Julian had asked me, and delighted that he had such faith in my people management and negotiation skills.

'It won't be an easy job,' he stressed. 'It's a huge operation: there are around a hundred people in each of the companies, and it will take a lot of wheeling and dealing to keep it on an even keel.'

There would be a lot of travel. 'You'll probably need to think about it,' he said.

At the time, I was negotiating with a theatre company that wanted me on board for a new project. I was currently trying to talk up my fee. By contrast, *Riverdance* was offering what seemed to me a small fortune. I talked it all through with Miriam, and she agreed that this really was too great an opportunity to miss.

With the birth of our two children, Hannah in 1993 and Loughlin in 1996, we had decided to move to the country. There was a place for sale in Lacken, west Wicklow, which belonged to family friends. It was essentially a holiday getaway – a chalet on a six-acre plot – but it had spectacular views overlooking the Blessington Lakes.

We had visited our friends for a weekend or two and loved the place for its peace and serenity. I was in Australia when it came up for sale and was somewhat surprised to learn, on my return, that Miriam had put in an offer. Surprised, but pleased. Much as we'd liked living in Rathmines – certainly it was convenient – we didn't feel it was the best place to bring up children. The country seemed a much better proposition.

We sold our Rathmines house for a sizeable profit, and moved in. The idea was to build a substantial wooden house on the land just as soon as we could get the money together.

'Think of the potential of this land,' Miriam had said as we looked around at what was basically a wilderness. 'I can do so much with this.'

And she did! While we were all camping in the chalet she got busy planting seeds, and in no time was serving up fresh vegetables from the garden. We bought some hens too and, eventually, a couple of pigs. It didn't come as a surprise when *The Irish Times* featured us in the property section, likening us to Tom and Barbara Good from the BBC comedy *The Good Life*.

This new job offer meant that we could build our house without delay. We both agreed that *that* was more than worth a few sacrifices.

From the start, the job with *Riverdance* was all-consuming. I was inundated with this great wash of emails flooding in day and night, all demanding tricky and complex negotiations with company members, with the crew, and with the young dancers.

'The problem,' Julian had explained, 'is that when we started out we didn't foresee the global popularity of *Riverdance*. We assumed it would have its run at the Point and that would be it. Everything was done more or less with a spit and a handshake, and maybe the odd letter, but now we need to put a shape on it. With your legal background, knowledge of the theatre world and reputation for fairness, I can't imagine a better man for the job.'

He reminded me of the time we had worked together in the theatre festival. 'I remember you as Box Office Manager,' he said. 'And I know how good you are under pressure. I know that you'll bring a sense of calm.'

There were so many different groupings on the show. There were, of course, Irish dancers, singers and set design-ers needed with the launch of the original idea, but when the show expanded, Russian dancers and Flamenco dancers were brought on board too, and I was to set a rate for each grouping.

The Dublin office was in a mews in Hatch Street. Julian and I occupied the top floor, with the rest of the team on the floor below us. I'd be frantically typing, feeling I was against the clock as the pile of paper grew beside me. The team, working below us, claimed to know when I'd had a particularly fretful day. The minute they saw me they'd say, 'Well, you've had a busy morning' or, 'A bit quieter today, I hear?'

When, bemused, I asked Julian how they always seemed to guess this right, he roared with laughter. 'It's your foot tapping, Ronan.'

'My foot tapping?' What *was* he talking about?

I hadn't realised it, but my feet tapped in time with my hands as I typed. Nobody had pointed it out before, but it was, Julian insisted, the case.

'And the faster you type, the faster and louder the tapping.'

'And they hear it through the ceiling?'

He nodded sagely. 'Apparently so!'

With the amount of travelling we – but especially Julian – were doing, and with the companies ever growing, we agreed that we needed a General Manager. We hired Ciarán Walsh to come on board, a man working in the world of theatre whom we both knew and respected highly. I became Director of Operations, a role that demanded more travel.

I would greet the teams at the start of the tour and sort out the initial problems, of which there were many. For example the set builders, tasked with the 'get in and get out' – a theatre term for putting up and taking down sets in a hurry – would complain about the one or two who weren't pulling their weight.

That wasn't the worst of it. There was the whole rock-and-roll madness, something I had never encountered before. And, particularly, there was the rivalry and clashing of egos between the lead dancers of the various companies.

We always seemed to be one step behind, struggling to keep order. When a friend asked me to describe what the *Riverdance* machine was like I said, 'It's a thundering juggernaut hurtling down the road while we, the managers, are hauling ourselves along the tarpaulin, inching towards the cab and desperately trying to get into the driving seat.'

We divided each tour into 'legs' of between two and five months. These would be separated by a rest break. The job of hiring and firing could be particularly harrowing. Thanks to my law degree I was used to sorting out contracts, indeed I had often been brought in by various theatre companies to help them secure actors. I was seen as a level-headed, fair individual who could distinguish what was my colleagues' needless worries were, in order to concentrate on the important issues. Because of this, the job of negotiating fees was second nature to me. The problem was that some of the crew, anxious to mark their superior pedigree, insisted on going to the top and dealing with Julian Erskine, instead of with me.

It wasn't just hiring and firing that consumed me. The emails pinging in each day could cover a myriad of issues. Some people, who wanted an instant solution, came knocking at my door. A dancer might limp into my office complaining of an injured foot, or a crew member might storm in saying an element of the scenery or lighting was not working the way it should. Most of these issues could be dealt with swiftly by simply handing out money. But you had to weigh it all up carefully, and work out calmly what was the best thing to do.

Having changed the face of Irish dancing in Ireland, *Riverdance* had opened up amazing opportunities for the young dancers who were part of it. They were earning really good money, but being so young – many were still in their teens – they caused me a particular headache.

Some of them had not been out of Ireland before, and so relished their independence. A few let it go to their heads. Although they were excellent dancers – they had to be to deal with the demanding choreography – they weren't familiar with the world of theatre. I lost count of the times I'd be called in to deal with yet another breach of discipline.

I'd say, 'Your dancing is excellent. No one is disputing that, but you need to take responsibility as a member of this company. If you want to remain working here, you're going to have to improve your timekeeping.'

Shamefaced, they'd say that they would. But dealing with many reoffenders, I'd press the point home.

'You're going to have to curtail your social life,' I'd say. 'Because if things don't improve, we're going to have to let you go.'

Sometimes the unaccustomed lifestyle would cause a dancer to put on a bit of weight. They had to be talked to or written to, but obviously a great deal of tact was required. As the member of the management team most known for diplomacy, these letters generally became my responsibility.

Being employed by the company gave the dancers great kudos. It also gave them high expectations and a heightened sense of self-entitlement. I might get a fax from Tokyo saying, 'My hotel room is terrible! If you don't organise a better one for me, I'm leaving on Friday.'

Disgruntlement could be catching. At one stage we had a series of complaints from the girls saying the rooms weren't up to scratch, and we agreed on a compromise. I said, 'If you're not happy here, we'll give you the money the room cost us and you can arrange your own accommodation.'

Happily agreeing, the dancers often chose much cheaper accommodation and pocketed the difference. Or, in one extreme incident, they lived in a caravan!

There was a certain disdain of the Dublin office. Sometimes the dancers, wanting something, would bypass me and approach John McColgan directly. Meeting him by chance, they'd ask him if they could have their own room.

He'd agree, because he wanted to see the girls happy. But I was responsible for the budgets. Annoyed, I'd check it out with John. He'd say, 'Oh yes, I did agree,' and there was nothing I could do about it. These so-called 'car park deals' could be somewhat frustrating.

Dealing with all this I'd think back to my years in theatre, and especially to the days with TEAM, when the work was more important to all of us than the money. We loved what we were doing, and these girls never seemed to be satisfied.

'I don't understand them,' I said to Julian after another complaint about accommodation. 'These dancers don't know just how lucky they are! They have so little under-standing about how the world of entertainment works.'

Audience appetite for *Riverdance* continued unabated. The number of touring shows increased to meet the demand from all quarters of the world, reaching a maximum of five. The work became correspondingly intense. Each production employed a hundred people and, with time, we had learned to be more careful whom we employed.

It was wonderful working with Julian and Ciarán, and we turned out to be an effective team. We had great fun – there was always a lot of laughter. One Christmas party we went in fancy dress and, as Director of Operations, aping a surgeon, I turned up in scrubs with blood stains all over me.

I'm an enthusiastic dancer myself – I always have been – but that night my exuberance went too far. My dancing partner, the equally exuberant Teresa Lonergan, who was Julian Erskine's PA, was sent spinning across the floor dur-ing a lively jive session and ended up sprawled over the drum kit. I've never lived that one down.

The first time I went to New York, and being short of time, I walked into a burger bar for a quick supper. Looking around, I couldn't help noticing how attractive all the waitresses were. They were so amenable too. One of them sat on my knee and dipped my chips into mayonnaise for me, before popping them into my mouth. 'This is amazing,' I thought. And I'd always been told that New York Americans were brusque and inhospitable.

I told this to Julian. 'They're never as nice in Eddie Rocket's,' I said, talking of a burger restaurant in Dublin.

Giving me a quizzical look, Julian asked me what the burger joint was called.

'It was a place called Hooters,' I said. 'And I can highly recommend it.'

Julian laughed so hard that I thought he'd fall off his chair.

'What's so funny?' I asked, noticing that Ciarán was in stitches of laughter too.

'You're such an innocent, Ronan,' said Julian. 'Hooters is famous for its scantily clad, beautiful young female servers. Did you not notice the absence of male staff?'

'The servers *were* rather underdressed,' I said. 'And now that you mention it, I can't remember seeing any guys working there.'

'You do know what "hooters" means – what the word is slang for?' Julian could hardly get the words out he was laughing so hard.

I shook my head.

'Breasts,' he said. 'Hooters is a place where groups of guys go for a bit of craic. And most definitely *not* the kind of place you slip in for a quiet bite to eat on the way to work.'

I laughed. I had to. It seemed I really was an innocent abroad.

In the main, *Riverdance* was tough, intense work, and I saw my family less and less, but the time came when the systems worked well. There were good teams of people firmly in place to meet and manage the demand for the show, and it was then that I was offered another fresh challenge.

Eleven

The Pirate Queen

Now that *Riverdance* was running on well-oiled wheels, John and Moya were looking for a new challenge, so they began mounting various international productions under the banner of River Productions.

The main project was *The Pirate Queen*, based on the story of Grace O'Malley, a sixteenth-century Irish warrior queen. O'Malley was a notorious pirate, and conquered the English before coming face to face with Queen Elizabeth I. She is seen as an icon of international feminism. With the history, drama and sea battles of Grace's story, it seemed the perfect vehicle for a musical.

When they asked me to leave my role on *Riverdance* and work with them on this new production as Executive Producer, Development, I accepted the role with enthusiasm. Leaving nothing to chance, John and Moya approached the very best to work on the production. They brought on board Alain Boublil and Claude-Michel Schönberg, the composers responsible for *Les Misérables* and *Miss Saigon*.

Excitement around the production was palpable and infectious and I threw myself into the work, loving the exhilaration of this unexpected and rewarding opportunity.

Travelling to New York with Moya; furthering the negotiations with Boublil and Schönberg; coping with it all and working at my best, gave the greatest satisfaction, but Miriam watched all this with mounting anxiety. I was now rarely home and, when I was there, I was often too tired to do anything but sleep and eat.

Shortly after my trip to New York Miriam and I were invited, in a party of honoured guests, to attend the launch of *Riverdance* in Beijing. It was October 2003, and Mary McAleese was visiting following the successful visit of the Chinese Premier, Zhu Rongji, to Ireland the previous year. A hundred and seventy-four Irish businesspeople were there too, with the purpose of seeking opportunities and forging bonds.

We were picked up at the house in Lacken by a chauffeur-driven limo. Miriam sighed with contentment. 'We're leaving all the chores behind,' she said, settling back comfortably. We met the rest of the group in the Executive Lounge at Dublin Airport, and were soon relaxing into slagging and banter.

There were sightseeing trips. Walking around the Forbidden City, I found it hard to imagine the monastic lives lived here over the centuries. That day, with the pathways dense with commoners wandering freely, it had the atmosphere of a film set.

Gala night on 6 October was an extraordinary, uplifting evening. Miriam and I walked up the steps of the Great Hall of the People under an umbrella: rain pouring down, the Doric columns towering above us. 'Who would have thought Irish dance would bring us so far?' I said, thinking how bizarre and completely unpredictable the conjunction of my life with the greater path of history was. Inside, there hung a huge oil painting of Mao Zedong, grandly guiding the people into the hall he had built for them.

Taking our seats in that audience of six thousand, listening to the buzz of expectation, I wondered how the show would be received. I'd always heard that the Chinese are reticent people, but they visibly loved the show, giving it a foot-stomping standing ovation. *Riverdance* had stormed on to conquer yet another territory! Would *The Pirate Queen* enjoy similar success? I wondered, before dismissing the thought. Tonight was all about celebration.

We met Ireland's president Mary McAleese at the reception that followed the show, and she could not have been nicer. Congratulating me, somewhat mistakenly, on my part in the proceedings she commented, 'I like your suit.' And Miriam behind me said, 'I did that!'

'Well done!' Mary laughed. She hadn't a pretentious bone in her body. It made a wonderful end to a great week, full of craic.

After this wonderful interlude – and an ecstatic welcome home from the children – it was back to work with a vengeance.

I relished the challenge, but can't deny that my stress levels rose. And Miriam, watching this, called me to account.

'You'll have to slow down, Ronan,' she said. 'The children never see you, and they miss you. I hate to say it, but you're becoming a bit more like your father.'

This came as a hammer blow. But was she right? I'd accepted that I'd inherited my father's workaholism, but it was another matter to believe that I was making the same mistakes that he had. I thought about it and realised that yes, she did have a point. I did, in truth, recognise my father's behaviour in myself. I had spent my childhood wishing my father was more present in my life and now, at ages nine and six, my children were suffering the same fate.

But I couldn't worry about that now! Not when I had been offered this most exciting, prestigious role, one that was giving my family even more financial security than before. And besides, it's hard to break the habits of a lifetime. Miriam did not let the matter lie. With tenacious persistence she brought it up time and time again, insisting that I address my work-life balance and make the requisite changes before I burnt out altogether.

In February 2004 I had a spell of time at home. Being there with Miriam and engaging with my wonderful children made me look at my life in a more organic way.

By this time, Miriam had exchanged her career in acting for one in horticulture. She had been working happily in *Glenroe* for over a decade when, in 2001, RTÉ pulled the plug. This had come as a huge shock to the cast – viewing figures for the rural soap were still high – but Miriam, happy enough to change direction, took a degree in horticulture and was now working as a consultant.

Alongside this, she had developed an interest in felting. Specialising mainly in framed pictures, she displayed her work at galleries around Ireland, and in Burtown House, Athy.

I loved being with my family: with beautiful Hannah who would hug me spontaneously and say, 'You're the best daddy!' And funny, sweet Loughlin who loved regaling us all with a string of bad jokes.

Wanting to give my children every opportunity in life, I was taking them to drama classes each week. I'd glance at

Hannah as she chatted away beside me in the car and think, 'I could look at you all day!' I could barely believe that this beautiful young girl could be my daughter. And when Loughlin won an under-eight art competition in Wicklow, I swelled with pride. 'That's my boy,' I thought, delighted at this early show of talent.

Digging in the garden, relishing the strenuous physicality of it, I found my mind straying towards work. *The Pirate Queen* was continuing its slow, grand journey towards its launch, inching forwards in unstoppable progress. The success of the show carried huge import for my future career. It would have an impact both on any future work and on my material resources. It was a gamble, I knew that.

Lying in bed at night, thoughts chased around my mind in a shapeless glob of anxiety, all of them to do with my responsibilities to my family. I added them up in my mind: the house, school fees, future university fees, medical costs. Catching myself, I'd wonder how I'd become so narrow-minded and materially obsessed in middle age. What had happened to all my artistic ambitions, my Beckettian sensibilities, my street cred as a bohemian?

Yet had any of us realised what an arduous journey *The Pirate Queen* would turn out to be? It was a full six years from the time John and Moya first conceived the idea until it came to full fruition.

The duo was throwing everything into the new musical. They were convinced that it was going to be life-changing, such a massive hit that it would leave *Riverdance* shivering in the shade. In order to concentrate all their energy on this they were happy to receive a business proposal from Julian Erskine, and the Finance Director Padraig Wynne, that the

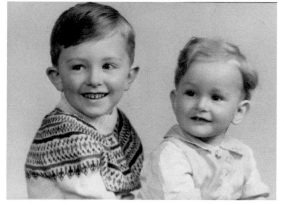

Julian, left, and me. Brothers, great pals, and partners in crime.

I spent many happy summers at Manch Farm in West Cork with my friend, Matthew. This was taken in 1975, when I was ten.

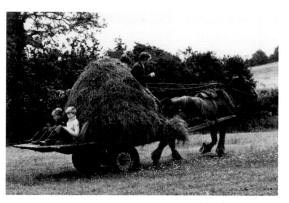

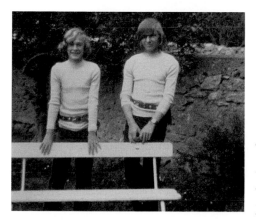

Two teenage blonds! Me and Julian, dressed to kill and posing shamelessly.

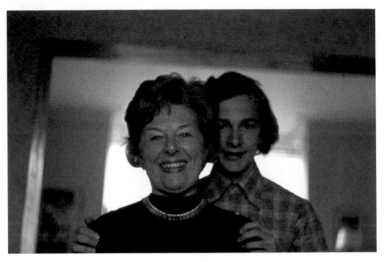

With my mother, the actress Beryl Fagan, who continued to tread the boards throughout her life.

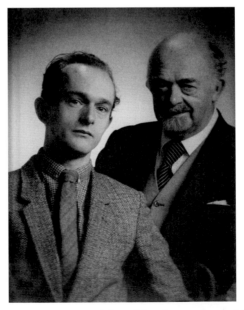

Taken for a newspaper article, this shows me with my dad, Brendan Smith, in the 1980s.

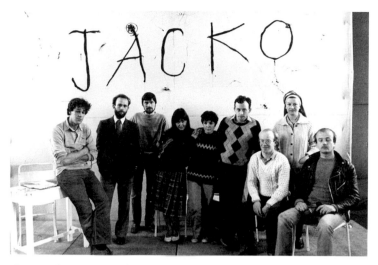

Cast and crew in *Jacko*, 1982, for TEAM theatre. I'm second from the left. (© Michael Foley)

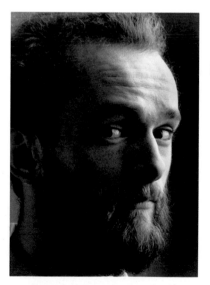

I grew a beard in 1990 to appear in *Macbeth*, directed by Martin Drury for the Second Age Theatre Company. Miriam appeared as Lady Macduff.

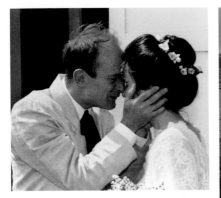

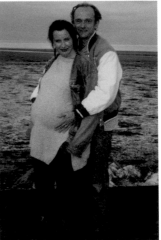

Miriam and I were married on May 26, 1990, a gloriously sunny, and intensely happy day.

In 1993 Miriam was pregnant with Hannah, our first child. Here we are on Sandymount Strand.

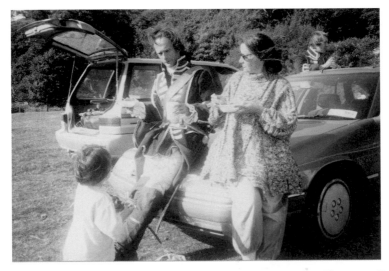

Picnic lunch with Miriam and Hannah during the filming of *Kidnapped*, at Luggala in the Wicklow mountains. I taught the actor, Armand Assante, how to fence, and was given the small part of Corporal in the TV movie.

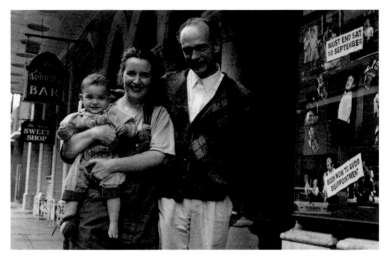

Miriam often brought Hannah to visit me at the Gaiety Theatre. In those days, I worked day and night!

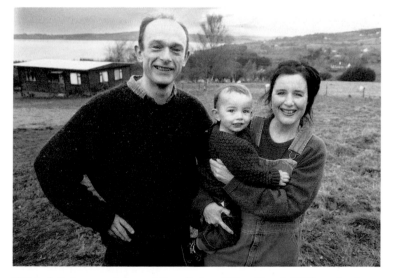

With Miriam and Loughlin, living 'The Good Life' at Lacken, before we built the house. The chalet is in the background. (© *The Irish Times*)

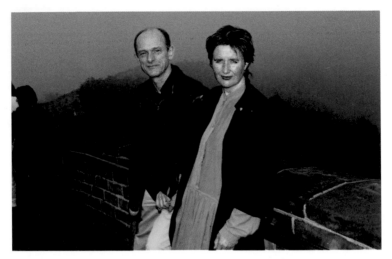

At the Great Wall of China, Beijing. We were there for the opening of *Riverdance*, in October 2003.

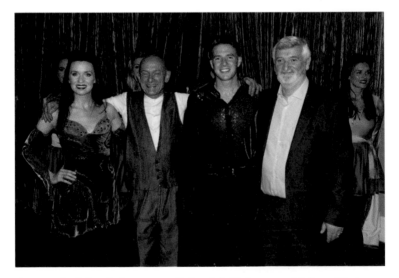

At my 60th birthday party, John McColgan and Moya Doherty surprised me with a performance by the Riverdance Flying Squad. Julian Erskine is on the right. (© John McColgan)

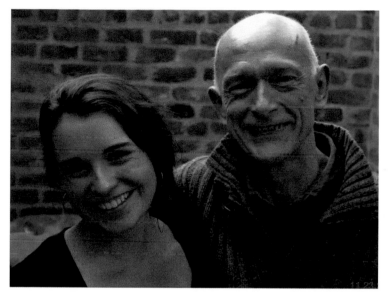

Hannah – my beautiful daughter.

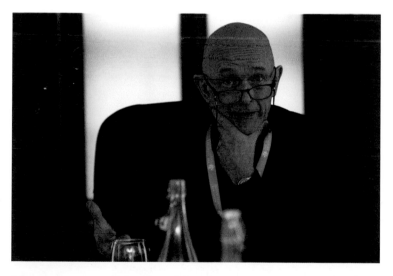

My advocacy work for the Alzheimer Society of Ireland has been important to me as a way to help spread awareness. Here I am chairing a focus group of people with dementia. (Courtesy of the Alzheimer Society of Ireland)

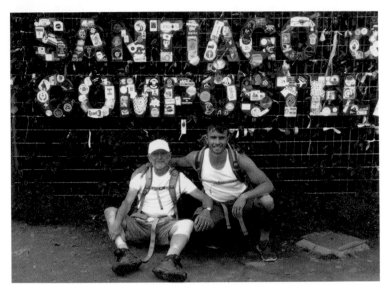

Father-son bonding in June 2018, when Loughlin and I walked the final stage of the Camino route in Spain.

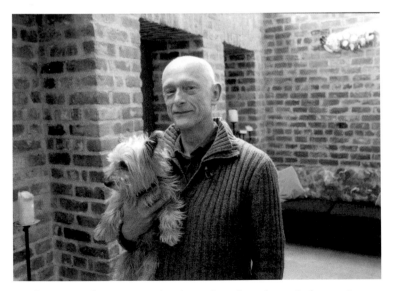

With Pepsi, the terrier who has played such a vital part in my Alzheimer's story, and helped me come up with my mantra.

management team from Abhann Productions would operate independently and continue to run *Riverdance* on a licence from Abhann.

To this end Julian, Padraig, and I set up Long Road Productions, along with Ciarán Walsh and accountant Gareth McCarthy. Julian and Ciarán would continue to drive *Riverdance*, but we would have the flexibility to produce our own shows and take on management projects for a range of clients. Julian Erskine was the Senior Executive Producer of Long Road and, as his second in command, my title was Executive Producer.

As part of the deal I continued my work with John and Moya, acting as their Executive Producer but under the Long Road Productions banner. This appealed to me, because however great the kudos was of working with John and Moya, I was essentially an employee.

We had early successes with Long Road. The most prominent was songwriter Shay Healy's new musical *The Wiremen*, an extravaganza about rural electrification. By 2006, with a raft of projects under our belts, the company was active enough to generate a good income for us all. These included many consultancies and management projects, including the opening and closing ceremonies for the Ryder Cup at the K Club in Kildare.

Much as I enjoyed the versatility of my work, my stress levels rose disproportionately. The initial excitement of *The Pirate Queen* – and it *had* been exciting, right from my first email to Boublil and Schönberg to the signing of the final agreement – was beginning to morph into anxiety.

In January *The Pirate Queen* was described in *Variety* magazine as a 'mega musical'. Expectations rose further. But I was feeling some disquiet. I was flying business class, living a life filled with glitz and glamour, but was the production going to be the runaway success that was being hyped? I was no longer sure.

In contrast to the bonhomie at the start of this venture, there were now nerves, fighting and stress. So many large reputations hung on this show's success. Trying to sort out the increasing number of problems, I felt I was at war with everyone. Again I yearned for the days of TEAM and that flexible, functional working environment. Yet that venture had not brought financial reward, and I needed that now. What was the answer?

On the other hand, this could well turn out to be the success everyone expected and, if that was the case, it would do my career no harm at all. It was a heady mixture, this drug of risk and possible fortune.

Miriam remained unhappy with my work obsession. Even my old friend Philip complained of it. We'd been meaning to meet up for ages, having left it longer than usual, and when we finally managed a lunch he told me firmly to turn off my Blackberry.

In August came some respite. We had 'The best holiday yet', according to Hannah and Loughlin. We were on the Greek island of Antiparos, and it was idyllic. I knew it, as we cycled and lazed around, and drank in that glorious Mediterranean sun. Yet I didn't relax. I couldn't. On the plane home, thinking all this through, I had to accept the truth. I was stressed.

It was one thing to know that, but quite another to do anything to remedy it. My days got even longer. I was working from 8 a.m. until 10 p.m. And if I *did* get home at a reasonable time, I was still on the phone until 10 p.m.

In October I flew to Chicago to watch the first dress rehearsal of *The Pirate Queen*. Sitting near Alain Boublil and Claude-Michel Schönberg, I was surprised to notice that they were astonishingly nervous. I watched the show dispassionately. At times I felt it was pretentious, overreaching stuff. Occasionally it seemed clumsy and lumbering, like a slighter version of *Les Misérables* and *Riverdance*. But at other times it was grand and impressive, then beautiful and moving. I came away feeling unsure.

After the first preview, however, audience reaction was good and I felt more hopeful. We all did. The feeling was, 'We have a show'. But our relief was short-lived. When the Chicago reviews came out, we were slated and dismissed. The welcome we had received in Chicago, and the audience acclaim, vanished in a puff of smoke.

Writing in the *Chicago Tribune* critic Chris Jones said, 'The earnest and epic but ill-ruddered and oft cartoonish voyage from the creators of *Les Misérables* and the producers of *Riverdance* is far from shipshape. How long its costly Irish sail will last in New York will depend upon the willingness of its creators to face potentially painful truths – beginning with a lack of clear commitment to the kind of legitimate, sophisticated, and above all, complex musical that has marked Alain Boublil and Claude-Michel Schönberg's glorious careers to date.'

Despite the disastrous reviews, the show did well in Chicago. The audiences liked it, so what had gone wrong? Thinking this over, I wondered if we had all given Alain Boublil and Claude-Michel Schönberg too much respect, their record of success had meant it was impossible to challenge them. Because the truth, I felt, was that the story of the musical was unclear and the characters failed to engage.

John and Moya took the reviews to heart and in the new year, deciding to tweak and improve the production, they brought in new creatives. Just as well, as the advance ticket sales in New York were disappointing. After those Chicago reviews, the market seemed to be adopting a wait-and-see approach.

Meanwhile, in my role as Executive Producer with Long Road Productions I went to a rehearsal of *I, Keano*, a comedy musical play about Roy Keane's travails in the 2002 FIFA World Cup. Watching the actors, feeling their down-to-earth enjoyment, I realised I missed Dublin theatre. Wasn't this what theatre was meant to be about? People simply enjoying themselves? It was a funny play and felt well worth doing. The evening had done me good. It highlighted how cynical I was becoming about my work.

In my day job I was feeling spare. I was flying out to New York business class – all expenses paid – in order to impose order on the enterprise, yet I had to trust that the creative team was up to the job. The sad truth was that they were in charge of my financial future.

The close of winter saw me in a bad and lonely place. Julian Erskine was away with the still enormously successful *Riverdance*, which was continuing to keep the Long Road coffers well stocked. That left the responsibility for the running of *I, Keano* firmly on my shoulders and, meanwhile, my worries about *The Pirate Queen* were intensifying. It didn't help that Miriam, burdened with the responsibility of taking sole care of our children, was feeling abandoned.

One day, cycling in the gym in a frantic effort to relieve my stress, I caught myself again copying my father's often uttered, 'Poor Brennie,' by muttering, 'Poor Ron-ie.' How had it come to this?

On my next trip to New York, *The Pirate Queen* had vastly improved, the story was now clear and understandable. That was good. And yet. I just wasn't sure how interesting it was. The music was grand and soaring, but not fresh. The staging and dancing were lively and ever-changing, but I wasn't sure how original they were. The costumes, sets and effects were sumptuous, but I'm not sure how impressive they were. The audience stood at the end, but I'm not sure how passionately. Would the show have legs?

I was unsure whether to look forward to the opening or dread it. The show, I felt, might not now be a failure. But even if it was the next step up – considered mediocre – that was a joyless prospect. I thought back to my excitement all that time ago and felt a hint of nostalgia.

The show finally opened on Broadway on 5 April 2007, and Miriam came over for it. The performance seemed to go well. We were all cautiously optimistic and gathered for the party with a sense of hope – hope that was dashed when the papers arrived. The only positive remarks were that the lavish sets and lighting were admired, but the multitude of lashings felt hard to take.

The New York Times concluded that, 'Everything blurs into what feels like the aimless milling of a crowd on a carnival midway. The operating theory behind *The Pirate Queen* would appear to be taken from an appropriately ocean-themed bit of zoology: if, like a shark, it never stops moving, then it will stay alive. The optimism is misplaced.'

If that was bad, Jacques Le Sourd of *The Journal News* was even more scathing, saying the script was like 'a comic book for 5-year-olds'.

The sense of disappointment was palpable. John and Moya were deeply shocked at the blistering nature of the reviews. And it wasn't just the two I've quoted, the papers were unanimous and extreme. There was nothing to say. The after-party emptied quickly.

As we went back to the hotel I was thinking of all those highs and lows of the past five years. Five years! Five years of work, of speculating and planning; five years of dreaming, of anticipating an enthusiastic reception, lay shattered. But was it devoid of *any* merit? Could we have got it so completely wrong?

One critic described it as self-congratulatory. How, I wondered, could music be self-congratulatory? Whatever, it was done. It was a nightmare. I tossed and turned, unable to sleep. Who would employ me now?

Meeting John and Moya the following day, I found them in fighting mode, joking and laughing. 'We won't take this lying down. We'll fight the critics. It's been done before. Look at *Wicked* and *Les Misérables*! The critics haven't prevented those shows from becoming phenomenal successes.' I hoped, without much conviction, that they were right.

Three days later reality had hit. The best we could hope for, it appeared, was a run of a couple of months. Home again, the dismal experience had me muddling along and watching as the vessel that had promised so much fought for its very survival. When I showed my management face in Limerick at the closing performance and party for *I, Keano*, I found myself pondering on the past, nostalgic for that time when I belonged with a cheery company of actors. Management had bought me material wealth, but it had also brought a sense of isolation.

After just eighty-five performances, *The Pirate Queen* sank. It closed on 17 June. What did this latest encounter with failure mean for me? It had been a stark reminder that the only reward of a commercial venture is profit. If you don't make a profit, there is no other compensation. This venture was devoid of social purpose, and about as far away from my beginnings with TEAM as it was possible to be. I craved a sense of worth, but there's a problem with that craving. Worth doesn't pay.

I was talking through this dilemma and the stresses of dealing with professional grief over lunch with friends. And listening, my old buddy Martin Drury professed surprise. Addressing the table he said, 'Ronan is so full of common sense, and handles everything with such equanimity – which, incidentally, Ronan, is what makes you so good at your job – that it's easy to forget that things do take a toll on him too.'

Thank goodness for Long Road Productions! In 2008 I was in charge of two main productions: *Magick Macabre*, for one of John and Moya's companies, River Productions, and *MacBecks*, which was our own creation and production. The latter was a Shakespeare-inspired musical based on the lives of David and Victoria Beckham. It was written by Gary Cooke and Malachy McKenna, and the hope was that it would find an international audience.

I had worries over both productions, worries that they were okay but not great, worries that we were overspending the budget. Again, work became a place of stress. And it wasn't simply the volume of work – I had dealt with that for most of my life – it was that I began to doubt my abilities and to take any perceived failure personally.

Home life, however, continued to provide a soothing sense of ease. The best weekends were like relaxing into a hot bath. Philip and his wife Una came over one Sunday and when Philip, staring out over the lake said, 'My God Ronan! Your beautiful wife, beautiful house and gorgeous kids – you must feel like you've won a jackpot!', I could only agree. And although I envied Philip his financial security, my jackpot suited me very well.

For all that, the autumn found me back chasing my tail. In addition to my work on the two productions I had taken on a report for the Arts Council, one for a project I felt, deep down, had little merit. I put off writing this, chastising myself for laziness. And meanwhile I had budgetary worries. What would happen, I wondered, if *Magick Macabre* failed to meet with success at the box office?

Up to this time, I had been 'hired out' by Long Road to work for River Productions. With the collapse of *The Pirate Queen*, *Magick Macabre* was the only remaining reason for River Productions to pay for my services. Would McColgan and Doherty still be able to afford me?

Matching my mood, the economic crash arrived and hung over the country like a pea-souper fog. And then the inevitable happened. John and Moya, disappointed with the sinking of *The Pirate Queen*, decided to take back the management of *Riverdance*, effectively cutting off the flow of revenue to Long Road from the still-popular production.

This spelled disaster: with the demise of the Celtic Tiger, Long Road's independent activity had pretty much dried up. There was a formidable atmosphere of caution around. Because the work that did come in wasn't sufficient to justify the extra costs involved in maintaining the company, we unanimously decided that we would be better off flying solo. We wound the company up and the five of us went our separate ways. Long Road Productions had been a brilliant employer for five lucrative years, but it turned out not to have been such a long road after all.

Twelve

Worrying Signs

Wanting security rather than run the risk of investing in theatrical projects, I operated as a gun for hire. Fortunately, I was able to generate a modest amount of professional work. At the start I concentrated on freelance management contracts for theatre shows, working with producer Noel Pearson and others. It was enjoyable work, but left me with too much time to spare and not enough income. Deciding to branch out, I began to seek out work in more general arts management consultancy. My experience with children's cultural centre The Ark, along with other boards I'd served on, meant this was a viable option.

It worked. Many opportunities presented themselves. They proved to be varied and engaging, less pressured than the theatre work and, crucially, required less of my time. I could do much of the work from home, thus cutting out the hours spent commuting.

Miriam was pleased. After all the years of sending me off and welcoming me home; of worrying about my workaholic tendencies; of managing the children and the house virtually single-handedly; of saying, 'There's more to life than work,' when my Blackberry interrupted dinner, she saw that I'd finally got the message. I was around, and able to pull my weight.

But had I left it too late? Back in the autumn of 2008 I had begun to experience random, sporadic and uncharacteristic lapses in attention and memory. I had put these slips down to my mood, and the anxiety about work. With work stress lessened, surely all would return to normal.

It hadn't. The rot had settled in. And it brought back, starkly, recollections of my father and his early issues with memory. Surely I wasn't going down the same path that he had? I couldn't be!

I went to London on a routine business trip and on the plane home, wanting to work on the journey, I realised that my briefcase was no longer in my possession. It contained important papers, along with my diary. Horrified, I realised I had left it in a coffee shop. Not only was I worried about the loss, I was terrified of the implication of it. However, I tried to keep my fears to myself. I did *not* want to worry Miriam needlessly.

But I couldn't hide it from her. She had been watching me. And towards the end of September 2009, when I'd taken our terrier Pepsi for a walk down to the lake, and got home to find the house full of lunch guests – guests I'd forgotten we had invited – she waited until everyone had departed, and then she spoke out.

'This is happening too often,' she said, following me into my office, where I'd escaped to get on with some paperwork. I mumbled an apology and said that I hadn't really forgotten, but the walk had taken longer than I'd expected it to. She wasn't fooled.

'Ronan. Either you don't care enough to remember anything – or you're getting Alzheimer's.'

'I wish you wouldn't say things like that.' I snapped out the words automatically, but the Alzheimer's reference had hit the mark.

We stared at each other in an uneasy silence.

'Well,' she said, 'what do you think is causing it? This memory loss?' She spoke gently now, the anger having fizzled away.

'I don't know,' I said. 'It could be because I'm worried, anxious even. I'm not in great mental shape.'

She shrugged and said, 'Maybe not. But Ronan, you had noticed?'

'What? That it's becoming a pattern?'

She nodded. 'And that perhaps it's getting worse?'

I stared at her. And spoke the truth I had never admitted to myself. 'I've been logging it,' I said. 'The lapses. For a month or two now.'

She looked at me, wide-eyed.

'Oh, it's nothing major,' I said, to lessen the impact of my words. 'I'm talking about small omissions: blanks, names I know well going mysteriously missing. But Miriam that's not so unusual – not at my age.'

She raised her eyebrows. 'At your age? Ronan, you're only fifty-two.'

'Yes, but Julian has these moments too, forgetting names,' I said, talking of my brother who is two years older than me. 'He told me. It's just senior moments, surely? They're bound to creep up on us all in some form.'

Miriam let it go. But I hadn't fooled her any more than I'd fooled myself. Something was definitely wrong and I could no longer deny it. I didn't sleep that night, nor for the few nights after that. I was wondering if Alzheimer's was genetic. I hadn't thought so but, remembering that my father's mother had apparently gone 'a bit funny' towards the end, I wondered if I was programmed to get this awful disease. And if Julian was getting it alongside me.

Worrying about it wasn't going to get me anywhere, so I decided to let the practical side of me take over. I needed to plan for the possibility of Alzheimer's, and straight away, so that if the very worst thing happened my family would not be left in crisis.

We didn't mention the 'A' word for some time after that. And although I still watched myself, and still lay in bed fraught with worry, a part of me didn't accept that my forgetfulness was a problem. I managed well at work, didn't I? Nobody there had a clue that there was anything wrong. And besides, I didn't believe that Alzheimer's *was* genetic. I had never heard that it was, and surely I would have when I was working with the Alzheimer's Society in their fledgling years, way back in the 1980s? It's true I hadn't kept up with advances in science since, but surely I would have been aware of something so fundamental?

The truth is that I had turned my back on Alzheimer's. I had hoped never to have to engage with it again. I hung on to the possibility that this particular kind of anxiety, at this particular time in 2009, might still have arisen solely out of a depression caused by circumstance. Because the anxiety had not gone away, it had intensified.

And in truth the situation did not get rapidly worse, at least if it did we both managed to live with it, and keep our worries to ourselves. The pattern continued as it had begun, occasional incidents followed one after another. They were small in themselves, just minor dysfunctions of memory that had little significant consequence. However, these incidents did affect me. I began to work from home more, taking any excuse to do so. I thought of this as 'hiding in the hills'. Over time I became less and less inclined to leave the house. And this, inevitably, had a knock-on effect in my professional life.

I was no longer pursuing new work contracts with any real vigour. But this lethargy could be some form of depression, couldn't it? Wasn't that, logically, the most likely reason? It was natural, I reasoned, with the fluctuations and failures of the past few years of work, and the disappointment around both *The Pirate Queen* and Long Road Productions.

And then there was my age. Who is to say that I wasn't merely suffering from some kind of middle-aged angst? Maybe it was a chemical thing and would be put right by some kind of hormone therapy. Whatever the reason, my self-confidence was taking a serious battering and I was struggling to recognise myself. I was changing and I did not like it, did not like it at all.

Miriam noticed the decline in my mood. We talked things over and she said, 'Ronan. Why don't you see a psychotherapist?'

Agreeing, I made an appointment to see one in October 2012. The psychotherapist was good. He gave me some very sound and practical advice. He said, 'Visit the rooms in your psyche, including all the ones you don't like to visit, the ones you find uncomfortable. Just sit with them for a while.'

I nodded, agreeing that I would try it.

'They become less powerful with familiarity,' he said.

I did as he asked, and he was right. They do. It was both useful and powerful advice, and helped me to regain some greater degree of composure.

In November 2012 I was busy on The Gaiety Theatre pantomime production. As the Line Producer, I was responsible for managing the production process. This could be an arduous and complicated task. There are a lot of people needed to deliver the show and therefore a lot of organisation required to get all the elements in place and delivered.

It needed all my focus, and I made a deliberate effort to forget all my agonising about the future. I concentrated fully on the job in hand and nothing else. I would simply do the job to the best of my ability.

And if I was acutely conscious of the gap between the controlled calm I was trying to project and the contrasting reality of my interior stressed state, it seems that I got away with it. Nobody at work ever noticed anything amiss. I gave them no reason to.

It was one thing to keep up this façade amongst my colleagues in The Gaiety, but quite another to present an engaged normality at home. And in December, with the work on the pantomime going full tilt, I coped by becoming passive when I was away from it. How else would I have the energy for those essential tasks?

Miriam put up with this – I suppose she was used to it – until the evening when she asked me to talk to Loughlin about a problem he had at school.

'He'll listen to you,' she said.

I agreed to chat to him – I really meant to – but hadn't yet done so two days later. But when Miriam said, 'Have you talked to Loughlin?' I said, 'Yes of course I have.'

I don't know why I lied. I suppose it was simply to avoid a reprimand from Miriam, but of course my lie was revealed. She was furious, and I can't say I blame her.

'I ask you to do this one tiny thing,' she said. 'And you not only let me down, you lie about it. Ronan, what's happening?'

'I'm really sorry,' I said. And I meant it. I felt both foolish and diminished. I muttered something about the stress at work, something Miriam was well used to hearing, but the truth was I was running scared.

In time I *did* talk to him about school and about his future. Then I decided to put my thoughts into words. I wrote him a letter. Stressing how much I loved him, and how watching him develop skills and talents filled me with pride, I handed on a piece of advice. He was to follow his dream, whatever that might be. If he did that, I wrote, he would have my and his mother's utmost support. This came in part from the frustrations I had, that acting had not remained at the forefront of my career.

'My advice to you,' I wrote, 'is to carry your talent, whatever it is. Carry it lightly, without arrogance; expose it only to let it be available to others, but don't crow about it, or demand admiration.'

That is the essence of my philosophy – it's something I have always tried to live by. The only problem was that now I was beginning to wonder if I still possessed any talent. And that scared me.

I was wondering how I'd get through Christmas, but it was lovely. Miriam's son Brian was visiting from Finland, where he now lived, and Miriam surprised me on Christmas Day.

'Your present is outside, Ronan,' she said.

We stepped outside and there, with red ribbons round their necks, were two donkeys. I'd been talking about getting some for a considerable time and was delighted with the gift.

As 2012 rolled into 2013, the pantomime pressure eased. It was back to arts management consultancy work, something that was well within my capacity, so my stress levels evened out again. When I signed a major contract with the Science Gallery, based in Trinity College Dublin, I was pleased. I was employed as a temporary replacement General Manager covering maternity leave, and didn't expect it to present any difficulties. But I was wrong.

The Science Gallery, I soon realised, was a very ambitious organisation, and it was driving an expansionist agenda. Once I would have loved that, it was reminiscent of my early days with *Riverdance*. There was that same high-octane energy, the same ambition, with lots of excitement and drive. All of this created a dynamic and thrusting atmosphere.

But time had moved on since *Riverdance*, and my capacity for excitement had been left behind along with my confidence and, indeed, my competence. I was out of step and struggling to deliver. For a while I carried on, thinking of the other times when an exciting challenge had spilled over into stress – a common occurrence for anyone in my line of work, since the line between the two was often a thin one.

But one morning, arriving early and before all my colleagues in order to get ahead and prepare for a meeting, things came to a head. I was collating papers into folders for each of the six attendees. A simple task. One a child could do. Yet I kept making mistakes, in fact I kept repeating the same mistake.

I couldn't understand why and, shaking my head, I had a good talk to myself. 'Just get it together, will you,' I muttered, as I took stock and started again. It didn't work. Another mistake. I slowed down and tried yet again.

And got it wrong. Then I sat back, breathed hard, and had a good think.

Why was this happening, and with such a simple task? I realised with dismay that this was a real dysfunction. I had to acknowledge it. Something wasn't right. And then it hit me. Hard. Right in the gut. I was acting exactly the way my father had.

Sitting there quietly, with a sick feeling in my stomach, I remembered that day I walked into my father's office and found him aimlessly ransacking sheaves of paper. Clearly frustrated, he had been tossing them hither and yon. It had been the moment I had accepted, once and for all, that all the fears I'd nursed about my father's capacity were true. He had a problem. And so, now, did I.

I sat at my desk and made myself breathe slowly and deliberately. In this way I calmed myself down and, with some difficulty, disciplined myself. I would *not* step into my father's shoes. He had been stubborn in his insistence that nothing was wrong; I would face up to this. I would no longer deny that this was happening. I would take action. The decision made, I relaxed, and finally completed the simple task.

I got through the day somehow. And when I got home, I told Miriam what had happened. 'It was terrifying,' I said. 'I'm like my father. I recognised him in myself.'

I'd been dreading telling her, worrying about her possible reaction, but of course there had been no need. She gave me a hug of support and said we'd manage it all together. The weight of worry lifted.

'I've been worried about you, Ronan,' she said. 'For months now. I've seen the signs too.'

'Of dementia?'

She demurred and said, 'Possible early signs, but nothing can be definite until you've seen an expert.'

'For a diagnosis?' I said, feeling a bit queasy at the thought.

She nodded. 'It makes sense.'

'No,' I said, turning away from her. 'That surely isn't necessary. Not for a while, anyway.'

This was too much. Too blunt. I wanted to equivocate. To duck and dive as I had done so often before. I truly hated the prospect, hated this possible imposition into my life. I was, quite simply, running scared.

This time Miriam didn't let me away with it. She persisted in telling me her worries, pointing out concrete behaviours that had led to those concerns. 'These memory lapses are real, Ronan,' she said. 'They require action. It may not be Alzheimer's, but if the worst happens, and it is, it would be best to have a diagnosis. And to have it early. Then we'll know what we're dealing with.'

'That's true, I suppose,' I spoke grudgingly.

'And Ronan, then you can have some treatment,' she said. 'There may well be a drug to remedy this.'

Reluctantly, I agreed. I would go for a test. Having given her my agreement, I felt lighter. There was real comfort in that acceptance. I slept well, and woke thinking yes, this has to be done. Miriam is right. It was that simple.

Except that, somehow, it wasn't at all simple. Making up our minds to do the test, and acting on the decision, are two distinctly different things. We were busy. Busy with work, life and our family. I was coping well enough, day to day. Managing. At work, nobody noticed that anything was wrong. We coasted, keeping fear and denial at bay. But eventually we reached that point where it really, truly, *had* to be done.

I made contact with my GP and through him we pursued an appointment with a specialist for a formal clinical test. It came in February 2014, and Miriam and I went to the Memory Clinic in St James's Hospital. It was a tense affair. I'd guessed that the testing would be calibrated in such a way that even an entirely healthy and functioning person would fail a certain number of tests, so getting every answer correct wouldn't necessarily be expected of anyone.

It was, I suspected, a 'gradation' exercise to see where approximately on the scale you fell. And going through the test, I *did* have some failures. I knew it at once. Hard as that was to accept, I tried not to be discouraged. Putting the errors to the back of my mind, I kept myself on course. I don't know how long the test took, but it felt endless, and it was challenging enough simply to keep focused.

When finally it was finished, instead of feeling relief, I was overcome with anxiety. I'd never felt this bad after any academic exam. I tried to work out how many mistakes I had made, and to ascertain how many you could make and still escape a diagnosis of Alzheimer's.

I made eye contact with the nurse who had conducted the test. I willed her to comment, to give me some idea of how it had gone. When she failed to do this, I searched her face looking for clues. And found none. And while I understood her need for non-disclosure, and the correctness and appropriate formality of the proceedings, the child in me needed the immediate reassurance that I had done well, that everything was okay.

And like a child, I left the clinic with a sense of deep disappointment. Sensing my sombre mood, Miriam joined me in near silence. We found the car, gathered the change to pay the parking charge and went home, each lost in our own thoughts. What was the point of a post-mortem? What good would speculation be? Time would tell.

Thirteen

Diagnosis

The dreaded day arrived. It was 21 March 2014, three weeks after I'd taken the memory test, and Miriam and I were summoned to St James's Hospital to get the results. As we sat together in the waiting room I was filled with a sense of foreboding. Why had we been called back? Why hadn't they told us the result over the telephone? Did it mean this was bad news?

I looked across at Miriam, seeking reassurance. The sight of her in her sunshine-yellow coat normally lifted my mood, but not today. Caught unawares she looked as gloomy and as scared as I felt, but meeting my eye she smiled. The smile did not reach her frightened eyes.

'Mr Smith? Mr Ronan Smith?'

We stood, and the receptionist pointed to a door in the corner of the waiting room. We entered. The consultant looked up from behind her desk, and briefly smiled. Then she introduced us to the man sitting at the side of the room. 'He's the social worker,' she explained, before scanning the file of papers in front of her. I sensed Miriam stiffen and I thought, 'That's clinched it.' Why would he be here if there was no problem to be faced?

I don't remember all that the doctor said. It was hard to concentrate as she talked us through the results of the memory test. But I will never forget the eight words she concluded with. Looking up, making eye contact she said, 'Probable early stages of early-onset Alzheimer's disease.'

'Probable?' Miriam clutched at the word, but we were soon to learn that it was there as a mere formality. A rock-solid, empirical diagnosis can only be given at autopsy, once the patient has died. In Alzheimer's, as neurons are injured and die throughout the brain, connections between networks of neurons may break down and many brain regions begin to shrink. By the final stages this brain atrophy is widespread, causing significant loss of brain volume.

It's commonly known that, once a sufferer has reached the middle and late stages of the disease, the symptoms are self-evident. I knew that, and so did the doctor. *She* knew the nature of the Beast. She knew he was at my back now. And I felt his malevolent presence. Or the return of it, as I had encountered him before. I had seen him stalking my father, slowly and remorsefully, and he was now at my heels. Slam dunk, no wriggle room, no equivocation.

I didn't look at Miriam, but I could sense her beside me as she fought with the shock and the fear. And meanwhile the doctor talked on, telling us what would probably follow, and what we could and should do to deal with the situation. She was formal, careful with her words and used a low-key tone, which seemed at odds with the drama of the life-changing news she was imparting.

A bit of comfort might have been nice. But if I wanted sympathy, I was in the wrong place. The doctor didn't say, 'Ronan, I am terribly sorry,' and she never said, 'How are you feeling, Miriam?' It was straight down to business.

I don't suppose it was easy for her, either. She couldn't offer us hope, because there is no cure at present and no potential escape routes to be discussed. Nor were there any options for effective treatments or interventions. We just had to suck it up. It was everything that we had feared and now it had been confirmed.

'Ronan,' she said, pushing the notes away and rising from her chair. 'I'm going to take you upstairs now to the cardiac unit.'

'Cardiac?' Miriam looked at her questioningly.

'I have to run a cardiac stress test on Ronan,' she said as she walked ahead of me. 'It's part of what we do here.'

She put me on a treadmill and measured the rhythm of my heart. When we returned to her consulting room, it was clear that Miriam had been crying. She tried to smile, but her red eyes and the tissue scrunched in her fist gave her away.

For the next few minutes we sat, frozen in shock, as the social worker took centre stage. His spiel was about the practicalities. There were a lot of them, but the one that stood out concerned driving. 'You have to tell the state about your diagnosis,' he said. 'And let your insurance company know at once.' He pushed some forms across the desk. 'You'll have to get a special licence every second year.'

To give the man his due, he did then try to lessen the blow. 'What you have is a disability that can be managed,' he said and that, I suppose, was true, for the present at least. Did he deliberately avoid mentioning the long, slow decline into advanced senility? A decline I knew so intimately, having watched my father so closely all those years before.

My head was spinning as we walked along the corridor, hearing muffled conversation and laughter from the various doorways we passed. Silently following Miriam's yellow coat down the worn, marble-effect stairs, I was in freefall. The sun shone weakly as we reached the car park. Miriam stopped dead.

'What is it?'

'I have absolutely no idea where I left the car,' she said.

I laughed at the irony. And, of course, we soon remembered that it was across in the far corner. It was just the shock that had ambushed us.

Except that it wasn't really a shock. As we sat in the car, feeling the need to just get out of there, I acknowledged that I had expected this result. I think Miriam had too although, like me, she had been praying that she was mistaken. And now, the best we could do was take in the reality, keep strong and support one another.

'Oh my God the children, the children.' Miriam covered her face with her hands.

'I know,' I said. 'How are we going to tell them?' Her son Brian would be shielded from all this. At thirty-six, he now had a family of his own in Finland. But the others would be directly affected. Now twenty-one, Hannah was at university, living in Dublin and working hard for her finals, and Loughlin, at eighteen, had his Leaving Certificate coming up in just three months' time. 'We can't tell Hannah and Loughlin,' I said. 'Not yet.'

Miriam took a deep breath as she inserted the keys into the ignition and turned on the engine. 'There will be changes for all of us.' She pulled out of the parking space.

We came home to an empty house and were alone with our thoughts.

'We mustn't rush into anything,' said Miriam as we sat together drinking tea. 'Let's just assimilate this.'

It had been a sickening sucker punch, we agreed. Planning the next stage was going to take time.

The next day I woke early, and over a solitary breakfast, gave myself a talking to. I thought back to a scene in *The Year of the French*, a television film I had acted in near the start of my adult career. It was a co-production between RTÉ and a major French broadcaster and, watching as I waited for my own scene to be called, a line had caught my attention.

The French soldiers and the rebel Irish, having joined forces during the Rebellion of 1798, had just lost the last decisive battle. The superior English forces were chasing them and they were in chaos as they retreated, being either arrested or killed.

Scrambling to escape, they entered a village and came across a blacksmith who, angry and fearful, shouted out at them, 'Why did you come here? Why did you come through our village, bringing all this on us?'

Fleeing, one of the rebels said simply, 'Who promised you a safe passage through history?'

That phrase really stuck in my mind. I'd thought of it often and, that morning, eating my breakfast alone, it resonated as it never had before. No one had promised me a safe passage. From that moment I learned to avoid the phrase, 'Why me?' Instead I now try to live by, 'Why *not* me?' Alzheimer's can strike anybody.

I looked around the kitchen. Everything was familiar. I toasted bread, poached an egg and made coffee, just as I had the day before. (Unless, of course, I'd eaten baked beans then, I wasn't really sure.) The view down towards the lake took my breath away as the sun made it glimmer, just as it always did. Yet everything had changed.

I stood at the kitchen counter drinking the final dregs of my coffee and wondered how long it would be before I disappeared. Would I live to see my children settled? Would I bond with future grandchildren?

When would we tell the children? Miriam and I discussed that later in the day.

'Let's at least wait until their exams are over,' said Miriam, and I agreed.

When Hannah rang asking how I was, I found it difficult to chat to her. The secret had opened up a barrier between her and me. I hated the dishonesty, but I knew the time wasn't yet right. Hannah told me she was stressed about her upcoming exams. 'There's so much to learn,' she said. 'It's really tough.'

The last thing I wanted to do was to add to her burden, especially as I knew the horrendous stresses that were coming down the line. Thinking of my father, and the desperate strain his illness had caused me, made me question the randomness of Alzheimer's. How cruel to be assaulted by this disease twice in a lifetime, once as a support, and now in the starring role. Then again, I told myself, this is a random universe. There are large hunks of meteors, some larger than our Earth, hurtling unpredictably through space, any one of which might crash into our planet one day and end the entire experiment.

The day moved on. There was work to attend to: phone calls to be made, and Pepsi to be walked. As I wandered the lanes with the terrier, the winter sun on my face, I'd forget for a minute that my world had overturned. It was an effort to take in that I had, indeed, been given this horrendous diagnosis. It was really happening. Life continued, but there was this added extra factor. There was a complex terminal illness to absorb and respond to.

Over the next few days Miriam and I talked. And we cried. And howled. And we railed at the unfairness of the situation we found ourselves in. We talked about the day of the diagnosis, and of how coldly the whole experience had been handled. I told her of the Beast – the creature of darkness – who haunted all of my waking moments. 'It's malevolent,' I said. 'And it's coming to get me.'

'I know. I know.'

'But right now it's toying with me. It's like a cat not killing a mouse outright, but playing with it, letting it go, and then catching it again.'

Putting her arms round me from behind, she kissed me on the back of my neck.

'Are you okay?' I asked.

'Well, I have this constant image when I hit the pillow each night.' Pausing, she scanned my face, meditatively. 'You know I'm a nervous plane traveller, right?'

I nodded, thinking, well that's an understatement!

'It's like I boarded the plane that day with you, and we sat down, and everyone was comfortable, and you were telling me not to be nervous and that planes are safer than cars.'

'Which they are.'

She raised her eyebrows, and massaged my shoulders, before coming to sit down beside me. 'But then the captain comes on and says, "We're going to be on this plane for quite a while. And we're going to experience a little turbulence now and again. And the turbulence will continue, and it will get worse, and you won't be able to get off the plane. And in the end, it will get so bad that I'll crash the plane. You'll know it's happening, but you won't be able to get off."'

I stared at her, appalled.

'But *I'll* be here, Ronan,' she said. 'I'm *not* getting off.'

One afternoon, a few weeks after we had received the diagnosis, I was in my office working. I was on a phone call to The Gaiety when I heard this awful noise coming from the kitchen. It was primal, like an animal in pain. As I finished the call Miriam called out and said, 'Ronan, you have to come in. It's all over.'

I saw Hannah hunched over on the sofa. She was roaring, 'No! No! No! No! No!'

'You know?' I said.

Sniffing, she nodded, and I sat beside her, leaving Miriam to sit on her other side. The three of us were crying. 'We're so sorry,' said Miriam. 'So, so sorry.'

When she had calmed down Hannah said, 'I'm not going to take my finals.'

I was shocked. Miriam gave me a look which meant, 'Just leave it.'

Later, when Miriam and I were alone, I brought the matter up again. 'Hannah can't throw her life away,' I said. 'That just makes a bad situation worse.'

'It's okay,' said Miriam. 'She'll change her mind. I know she will. Hannah is a lot stronger than she thinks she is.' And she was right. Hannah took her degree in Social Policy at Trinity College and passed with flying colours.

I wondered how Hannah had learned the truth, and Miriam explained. She, Miriam, had been seeing a counsellor to help her learn how best to cope, and support me, and she'd borrowed a book called *Contented Dementia*. 'It's written by a lady who nursed her mum,' she said.

'It was in my bag, and my bag was here in the kitchen. I was putting on the kettle when Hannah appeared and said, "Mum, can I borrow your phone?" I said, "Yes, it's in my bag." I was standing here making tea, and when I turned around, Hannah had the book in her hand. She said, "Mum, what's this?"'

'So you told her?'

She shook her head. 'I bluffed. I said, "I have to do some research for the Samaritans." But Hannah said, "That's not true. It's not. Is it?" And I admitted, "No. It's not."'

She touched me lightly on the arm. 'I felt utterly sick. I thought, "Jesus Christ, it's too soon." And oh, Ronan! Her reaction!'

'I know,' I said. 'I heard her. Actually, I thought it was an animal.'

Miriam nodded. 'She threw the book on the floor, collapsed onto her knees and roared.'

'But Miriam, what now? Should we tell Loughlin?'

She shook her head. 'There's no need. Let him get through the Leaving Cert first.'

That was May. Loughlin sat his exams in June. After he finished them he went out to celebrate, but the next day he was sitting inside on the couch and we decided we could no longer delay. We sat down with him and Miriam said, 'We've got something to talk about. Ronan isn't well.'

Loughlin didn't look at us. His eyes were fixed firmly on the floor. Miriam touched his arm and said, 'Ronan has been diagnosed with Alzheimer's disease.'

He was silent. I hadn't expected the wild reaction we'd got from Hannah, but such passivity left me floored.

'Is there anything you want to ask?'

He shrugged. 'No.'

'Well, is there anything you want to say?'

'Well, I knew.'

'What?'

Loughlin looked up at last. 'It's not a surprise.'

I was dumbstruck and tried to work out who, of the small number of close friends we had confided in, could have let the secret out, but Miriam showed more composure.

'How did you know, darling?'

'I just had my suspicions. I've had them for a while now.'

He talked of a weekend two years earlier when I had taken him and a group of his school friends off on a three-day surfing break in Lahinch, Co. Clare. I'd been looking forward to some fatherly time with my son, and was all too aware that with my work commitments (or obsessions), occasions like this were rare.

At the time I was conscious of something not being right with my health, indeed it was after the first time Miriam had raised the topic with me, wondering if my occasional memory lapses and blanks might possibly be the start of Alzheimer's. I'd felt anxious about the trip, fretting excessively about the logistics, double- and triple-checking everything. This behaviour had made me feel like a stranger to myself, but the weekend had worked out well.

I had loved spending time with the boys, and it didn't bother me when I turned out to be pretty terrible at surfing. I only managed to stand twice, and then only for a few seconds. So what? I didn't care. It was the boys' enjoyment that mattered. I had cheered, genuinely pleased, as the teenagers glided past me, confident and exhilarated.

'I thought that weekend went well,' I said, puzzled and a little hurt.

He agreed that it had. 'But Dad, in the car going down, you asked James if he went down to the house often.'

'James? He's the one whose family owns the house we stayed in, isn't he?' I wondered where this was going.

'That's right. But you asked him the same question three times in the space of an hour,' he said. 'You'd completely forgotten that you'd already asked him. And then, when we were eating supper, you asked him another time.'

This shocked me. I had been completely unaware of it. 'I'm sorry,' I said. 'That must have been embarrassing for you.'

He denied that, but said he had been worried. 'I'd noticed before then that your memory wasn't great,' he said. 'There were times you forgot things, but I'd told myself that was part of your character, just who you are, and you had a lot of stuff going on. But that weekend I really started to worry. I thought, "Okay, this isn't just forgetful."

And besides,' he continued, 'your dad had Alzheimer's. I suppose I was always looking for signs.'

'Oh Loughlin!' Miriam was upset. 'That must've been really difficult for you – worrying and keeping it to yourself.'

'Well, I did tell my roommate at school,' he said. 'And he was really sympathetic.'

'Is that the lad whose father had cancer?'

'That's right. He was great. He listened and just said, "Well you could be right – who knows?"'

I was taken aback by his reaction, and by Hannah's. But I was glad that it was now all out in the open and we could share our thoughts and fears. There was no longer any need for secrecy: we could face the future as a family.

Fourteen

Coming to Terms

While Miriam and I were waiting for the 'right time' to tell the children, I had shared the news with my closest friends. Philip Lee was the first I confided in. A few days after my diagnosis I cycled over the Wicklow Gap, a beautiful route that winds through the Wicklow hills from the Blessington Lakes to Laragh, and he cycled to meet me from his home in Dalkey on the coast south of Dublin.

That was a big deal for Philip back then. He had just been through a traumatic cancer treatment, but was now, thankfully, in the clear. It was a beautiful, sunny spring Sunday, and being early I met few cars. But I was cycling with a heavy heart, dreading giving Philip the bad news.

We met just outside Glendalough, parking our bikes beside some army jeeps. 'This is going to be hard,' I thought. Still processing the news, I had been veering from grief to anger and back to grief again with the regularity of a metronome. There was no good way to share my news and I blurted it out without any preamble. Philip looked at me silently for a while, his eyes welling with tears. Then, slapping me on the shoulder, pulling himself together he said, 'Well, you've topped my health crisis!'

We hugged, and when we pulled apart noticed that a company of soldiers, in the mountains to perform some kind of exercise, were watching us with some bemusement. We entered Clodagh's café in an uncomfortable silence, but when we sat down with our coffee Philip took on his legal and business persona.

'Well, Ronan, you must fight the illness,' he said. 'I'm sure there are research trials, you know, experimental drugs you can try.' It was so like him to take a positive stance.

'Yes, yes,' I said, 'of course, I'll try anything. Well, anything within reason. But Philip, I've got to accept the diagnosis. And I'll have to work out how to deal with whatever happens next.'

He nodded, looking at me gravely.

'I owe it to my family,' I said. 'I have to construct some sort of order in my life, some sort of security.' Sipping my cooling coffee, I sighed. Just saying the words stripped away the lingering feelings of unreality. With Philip's help, I went through the practical steps that I would need to take.

I didn't mention my father, who had never accepted his diagnosis and who, through continuing to work, made life impossible for those around him. I didn't have to. Philip knew. He'd been around during those dark, difficult days.

When I got home I told Miriam how good it had felt, talking it all through with Philip.

'That's great, Ronan,' she said, continuing to chop fresh herbs from the garden as she prepared our dinner. 'But there's someone else you need to tell.'

'Julian?' I said, referring to my brother.

'Yes. He needs to know,' she said.

I knew she was right.

Back in 2009 when I first became conscious of my 'senior moments', I'd discussed it with Julian. Naturally anxious, he said that he too worried about himself. At the time he was stressed at work. Now working as an expert in IT, Julian had nothing in common with his GAA-mad workmates and he felt isolated. But would stress account for his moments of blankness, he pondered. Empathising, I said, 'It happens to us all. Things that used to leap along now limp along.'

We'd continued to mull it over, comparing ourselves with our contemporaries. Were we worse than them? Did we worry more? Probably. It was hard not to when we had seen first-hand the devastation dementia trails in its wake.

I rang him and we arranged to meet in KC Peaches in town for lunch. It's a good place to talk, not too loud, but with a little background noise to provide cover and enable him to react. Reminding him of that former conversation, I told him I'd had continuing difficulties at work. 'I went for tests,' I said, 'and I have news. I have probable early-onset Alzheimer's. I've had the diagnosis.' I shrugged and said, 'Just like Dad.'

He stared at me for a beat in silence and absolute stillness, then inhaled a sudden, shuddering, deep breath. We talked quietly, quickly focusing on the practicalities that could and should be addressed. At our parting, however, we both cried stutteringly and briefly, each trying to be strong for the other. The Beast was having a good day.

I met another close friend, Martin Drury, a few days later. When I rang asking to see him, he suggested we meet at the Arts Council offices on Mountjoy Square where he was working at the time. We had the building to ourselves, everyone else having left for the day, so it was very quiet.

I'd attended quite a few professional meetings there over the years, some of them challenging and difficult, but I'd have swapped the worst of them for the one I was now about to convene. There I was sitting opposite Martin, telling him that I was on a one-way journey into illness, increasing disability, confusion and, ultimately, utter dependency. I could see the shock in his eyes, and saw too the careful and considered calm he imposed on himself. His response to the news was immediate and heartfelt.

'I'll support you, Ronan, in any way I can,' he said. 'You can count on me.'

I was both touched and grateful, though not surprised. The conversation felt strangely slow, measured and very real. It was a good feeling: yet another strong block of support under my feet.

From that moment, the news began to leak out. It only took a day for Vincent Dempsey, an old friend and theatre colleague, to get in touch. He called to the house and we walked up the hillside above it while I talked through my feelings, as well as my initial plans for dealing with the diagnosis. All of these encounters and conversations steadied me in a very real and meaningful way.

The one person I had not yet told was Julian Erskine. Worried he would learn the news from somebody else, I had left several messages for him, but he had not responded. Miriam manged to contact him one morning and, hearing her voice, he apologised. 'I know, I know,' he said. 'Ronan has been trying to get in touch, I will get back to him, I promise. It's just that the schedule here on *Riverdance* has been crazy – even crazier than usual.'

She warned him that there was some bad news, and he arranged lunch for the two of us for the following day.

He has since proved to be the best ally and a constant, dear friend.

The strain of telling people, however, was beginning to tell. I wasn't sleeping and the emotional turmoil was wearing me out. After my lunch with Julian I felt, suddenly, bone weary. Seeing me yawning, Miriam suggested I should take an afternoon nap. 'I'll join you,' she said, telling me she was exhausted too.

'It's the future planning and speculating,' she said, as we lay together on our bed. 'It's so utterly terrifying.'

I nodded my agreement. My head was churning. I was coming down from the initial shock rush that had been protecting me somewhat. 'You know what,' I said. 'I just want to stop thinking about it.' I put my arms around her and drew her close. 'But mostly,' I muttered, 'I want it not to be real – not happening at all.'

We cried then, both of us, sharing our fear, our anger and our hurt. Then we talked. We started with the practicalities, discussing work, money and how our lives should change. I mentioned the social worker, remembering some of the things he had told us, and at once Miriam stiffened.

'What is it?' I asked.

'That man,' she said.

'The social worker?'

'Yes. Him. I could have killed him that day of the diagnosis.'

I looked at her, surprised. 'He was only doing his job, love. It wasn't his fault that the news was so bad.'

That's when she told me.

'You know when you went for that cardio test?'

'You mean the stress test? When I was on a treadmill?'

'That's right. Well, the social worker went off to get a glass of water for himself, and by the time he came back I was crying.'

'Well, that's understandable.'

'You'd think so, wouldn't you? But he said, "Is there something the matter?" And I looked at him, thinking of all the things I was having to face, and said, "Yes." And do you know what that man said, in his burr of a Scottish accent?'

'Tell me.'

'He said, "Well, you'd better pull yourself together, because Ronan is going to be coming down those stairs in a few minutes."'

'Oh God!'

'And that's when I wanted to kill him. I felt I had no support, and no permission to cry.'

Miriam and I have always had a strong, close marriage, and that mattered now more than ever. We still love each other deeply and I know I can rely utterly on Miriam's support. But I don't want to ruin her life, and I have to think of her future, as well as mine.

'Miriam,' I said, looking her in the eye and maintaining eye contact. 'We'll manage the practicalities as best we can. And we'll incorporate all those good and solid family members and friends, we'll accept their help and support through all of this.' I stroked her arm, then took both of her hands in mine.

'But there is this,' I continued.

'Yes?'

'If it *does* run to the point where I don't really know who is looking after me, I want you to feel free to have me minded in care.'

She shivered, and opened her mouth, about to speak.

I put my finger to her lips. 'And I want you to be very practical,' I said. 'I won't need a posh home. I won't need you to be spending money on something really expensive. I will be very happy in a state home, Miriam. I won't know where I am. So please promise me you will just be sensible.'

She looked appalled.

'I won't know the difference. And Miriam, this is important.' I squeezed her hands again. 'I love you. And I need to know, if and when the time comes, that you will take back your life for yourself. Please, please *promise* me that you will do that.'

She sighed deeply and glanced distractedly around the room. Then, shrugging, still not looking at me she muttered, 'Okay.'

'Could you say it more definitely?'

At last she met my gaze. And, taking a deep breath, she said, 'Ronan, I will do that. Yes, I promise.'

I think we both felt stronger and clearer after that conversation. When the very next day a close childhood friend, Matthew, arrived unannounced, I felt more able to cope. His wonderful family had embraced me back in our schooldays, letting me stay with them on their farm in West Cork each summer.

Appearing on the doorstep, he held his arms out for a hug and said, 'Surprise!' Little did he know that the surprise was on him! I thought of keeping quiet, for about a second, but I was too enmeshed in the heat from the moment of diagnosis to do anything but blurt out the truth. His reaction was immediate: acutely shocked, he expressed sorrow and support. Another pillar of strength was embedding.

The more people I told, the stronger I began to feel. I was beginning to realise that engagement and action helped me. Being real and honest about the illness was a positive thing for me: it could help me. In fact, the more real I could be, the better. 'This would be a good mental-health strategy for me,' I thought, and I decided to launch myself into exactly that.

Inevitably, these thoughts brought to mind my father who had never, to my knowledge, confided in anybody. Of course, those were different days, days when any kind of mental illness held the greatest stigma. But how different would the course of his illness have been, I wondered, had he chosen a more proactive role?

Thoughts of my father were ever-constant now, and old memories came hurtling back. And in reliving those memories, old hurts hit me anew. Pondering on the course my father's illness had taken, I projected my own future onto that which was in my father's past. It was not an edifying image.

Yet I knew, in truth, that I had options, opportunities and choices, ones that he had chosen not to pursue. I also had the benefit of the increased knowledge and understanding that the science had brought over the years. My journey was *not* going to be the same as his. But then again, each and every individual dementia journey is different.

I was on a mission. I would do everything in my power to learn all there was to know about the illness, and to take any action I could in order to slow its progress. And the first step was to re-engage with the Alzheimer Society of Ireland (ASI).

This wasn't only to learn of any possible treatments – although, of course, the hope of advancements was on my mind – it was also to find out what *I* could do for *them*.

I realised, with my history, I was uniquely placed to help them. If I offered to 'out' my diagnosis publicly, I could talk about the history I had with my father's experience of the illness and compare that with my approach to receiving a similar diagnosis. I contacted them, they were delighted with my ideas, and so it was that I became an advocate for the ASI.

But what about my career? I was aware that my current level of activity, giving rise to extreme stress, was proving untenable, but it was surely possible to keep up a level of professional work and do this in tandem with the advocacy work in the ASI?

It would mean an adjustment of my attitude towards work, I knew that too well! The buzz of multitasking and the drug of hyperactivity were off the agenda, that was for sure. Wishing to avoid the shock of going cold turkey, I decided to put in place a healthy balance of paid work and advocacy. I believed that keeping active – working with others in a purposeful way – would be beneficial to my health, especially as the advocacy work helped others.

I was lucky to have a choice. Often, when Alzheimer's comes calling, the result is immediate redundancy. Through ignorance and fear, employers tend to react in a knee-jerk way but, in truth, this overaction is rarely necessary. I believe there should be a legal requirement for companies to be more flexible and imaginative after an employee's diagnosis. Such societal attitudes contribute to a destructive secrecy and stigma around the condition. My hope is that people learn to be understanding and, on hearing of a friend's Alzheimer's diagnosis, keep their ears and minds open. If *they* face the situation, it makes it easier for the sufferer. They will then be able to discuss their condition and their fears for all it might entail. And while things are now considerably better than they were for my father back in the 1980s, there was still much to be done.

For once in my life, the precarious world I had chosen to work in, that of the arts, was paying dividends. My employers were flexible. I was able to continue with my work for The Gaiety Theatre pantomime along with some other productions, as the management was willing to negotiate a slightly adjusted work brief.

More importantly, I felt utterly comfortable there. I was working with a well-established team of people I both trusted and liked. It was almost like a family and I knew I could count on their understanding and support.

The advocacy work for the ASI proved a positive force in my life. In addition, becoming a member of the Irish Dementia Working Group (IDWG) – a group of people living with the condition that volunteers to assist the professional ASI staff – helped me to battle against the waves of hurt and anger that had accompanied my diagnosis. I felt that I was fighting back and giving the Beast a run for his money.

As members of the IDWG, we attended regular meetings to discuss our condition, comment and give on-the-ground feedback on 'The Living Condition'. In doing so, we helped inform the organisation's understanding of Alzheimer's and promoted their policy development.

Along with other members of the group I gave talks at a wide variety of meetings and events, sharing my experience of living with the condition. This further informed the society and became an important element of the strategies being advocated for.

There was, however, a downside to all this. In spending so much time talking of my condition – analysing and explaining it – I began to obsess about it, trying to estimate how long it would be before my deterioration became absolute. Would my experience mirror my father's, or would my proactive attitude delay the progress of my illness? Lying in bed I'd wonder about my father's journey, trying to remember any early signs. When *did* his illness actually start? How long had it been going on? He'd hidden it of course, so there was very little trail to follow, yet the obsession continued unabated.

And of course I did the one thing that doctors are always advising their patients not to do: I took to the internet and was overwhelmed with a deluge of information, little of it useful, even less of it encouraging.

What did I glean from it all? Not much that I did not already know. It confirmed that there was no effective cure at present; it stressed that the disease is terminal, but that the time frame is variable and uncertain. And it told me what the statistical range of that timeline was. I learned that I could expect to live between eight and twenty years before the disease killed me.

That statistic, being so vague, gave me little comfort. It was nothing more than idle speculation. As in all things Alzheimer's, it varies from individual to individual. And as such, my future remained an elusive mystery, and that mystery left me deeply distressed.

I'm a fastidious individual – a planner. I like to know where things stand so that I can settle my affairs. With this type of personality it's not surprising that this uncertainty caused an insidious undermining of my confidence. This was one of the Beast's teasing tactics, and it did not suit me at all.

During the years of my father's illness in the 1980s, the

unhelpful and histrionic name frequently given to the disease in the media was 'the living death'. It was perhaps a usable title for a horror movie, but it was singularly unhelpful in supporting people living with the diagnosis. It stuck in the head, however, and, once heard, played on repeat.

My previous Alzheimer's journey, with my father, often felt and still feels like a double-edged sword: useful to a point, but uncomfortably clinging and haunting at the same time. Speculating on how the late stages might be for me, what I came to hope for was simple: that I will be contented and agreeable for the sake of those who care for me. This is not something that I can guarantee to achieve, of course – the disease may find its own path – but I hope for it very much.

Absorbing the diagnosis is a strangely drawn-out thing. With no real road map to follow, no predictability, one is drawn to revisiting the experience of diagnosis as if it were not yet fully grasped. Although I accepted my diagnosis of being in the early stages of probable early-onset Alzheimer's, I couldn't imagine how it would feel as the disease shifted into the middle and late stages. They are a completely unknown experience for me, an impenetrable fog, so I am now effectively a stranger to my future self.

This is a very peculiar and uneasy place in which to find oneself. And it makes me more determined to ensure that Miriam understands she should care for me at home only as long as she wishes to. I keep repeating this instruction to her – emphasising that my present self is clear and determined about this. And this applies, whatever my mood and state, as my illness progresses.

'I won't understand the difference,' I tell her. 'If I am placid and agreeable in the final stages, I will be happy to be looked after in a decent residential care home. And if, God forbid, I become difficult and demanding, I will be perfectly all right in an acute care unit. My world will be my world, wherever it is.'

I have always gained great solace on my walks around the country lanes near our house. And Pepsi, the terrier we gave Loughlin for his sixth birthday, proved a calming companion. One morning not long after I had received the diagnosis, I was walking the dog by the lake, ruminating on how I would handle living with my condition. I decided I needed a strategy and concentrated on coming up with one.

I felt I needed to break down the response into a number of different areas, to lessen the feeling of one single, big, messy crisis that was turning my life on its head. There were the practical realities to be dealt with and to be prepared for: financial steps, legal steps, revising work planning, all directed to address the probable play-out over the next number of years. Then there was the opportunity to discover what appeared to be possible in altering my lifestyle to best combat the rate of progression of the disease. Finally, there was the need to encourage in myself the development of a positive attitude that would motivate me to continue addressing these challenges.

I came up with a mantra, one I continue to use. It's 'Prepare for the probable, work for the possible, and hope for the future'. It has helped me in many ways, offering practical solutions when life begins to feel overwhelming or when I lose heart. I often thank Pepsi for his part in this particularly fruitful walk.

Fifteen

Rolling with the Punches

My condition was now known to friends and to a few within the wider community and, while people were accepting, it was difficult to know how to respond to them when they asked earnestly, 'How *are* you?'

I came up with the phrase, 'I'm fighting the good fight.' That seemed like an appropriately breezy response and was an accurate picture, since most of the time, keeping positive, I was fighting the Beast happily enough.

It was not, however, the full picture. Living with Alzheimer's, for me, is a roller-coaster ride. I make a point of living in the moment – since looking ahead to what will inevitably come is not good for my mental health – and I roll with the punches. But there are times when a fog rolls slowly in, creeping up the shore, and sits heavily, obscuring everything.

Early in September on my habitual morning walk, I remembered giving some of my diaries to one of the PAs in Julian Erskine's office and asking her to edit them for me. But was that a memory or something I had dreamt? For several minutes I simply could not be sure. Then I realised that I would never have given a stranger a diary containing my innermost thoughts. How could I have imagined, even for a moment, that I would have?

I gazed over the lake lost in thought, as Pepsi raced around me, giving the occasional bark to remind me of his presence. It felt as if my memory was sliding on ice – lacking traction. A few days later, reversing out of our drive, I narrowly missed hitting a friend's jeep which was sitting near the gate. I'd known it was there. I had seen it and told myself a minute before that I had to be careful. And in that one minute, the memory had vanished. I had completely forgotten it was there.

At these times, all the positive health steps Miriam and I have put in place seemed futile. In this negative state, I believe that my physical exercise, my healthy diet and the cognitive exercises I carry out are sadly destined to failure. I see it all as misguided, foolish and desperate.

After I hit rock bottom, however, there is a strange and rather wonderful bounceback. And I can call a halt to the low mood as I consciously, and very deliberately, reconstruct a comeback. Positive again, I swear I will be able to prevent a return dip, yet it inevitably happens. I am stuck with it, lap after lap.

Much as I was enjoying my professional work, and recognising its worth for my ongoing cognition, I had, perhaps, taken on too much. A few months after my diagnosis I was involved, hands on, in two theatre productions: the annual panto at The Gaiety and the upcoming revival of *I, Keano*. Work was absorbing too much of my energy and capacity, sucking up all my time.

There I was in my rather shabby office at The Gaiety – a lonely place most of the time – tipping away at emails, handwriting to-do lists, working at a lamentably slow and inefficient pace. I had to double- and triple-check everything and, even so, mistakes slipped through. Digits mixed up in phone numbers, a date misplaced in a calendar appointment, small things that can have a disproportionate significance.

I took breaks, and wandered down Grafton Street for fresh air and a coffee from McDonald's. This was my treat. Wandering past the buskers, skirting around the crowds the best ones drew, being part of the pulsating life of this most vibrant shopping street for a minute or two gave me a much-needed boost.

In this autumn of 2014, none of my work was of the high-octane-stress variety. Gone were the glitzy glory days of the West End and Broadway, that was for sure! Yet certain stresses remained. I was still the breadwinner for my family, and the strain of it was taking its toll.

Miriam noticed this. And taking the initiative, she booked us an October weekend to Venice. Showing me the plane tickets she said, 'It's a gift. To us.'

I was grateful. It would be good to get away from this crisis that had overtaken our lives. And it was truly recuperative. From the moment we arrived into San Marco and saw the San Giorgio Maggiore across the water, the city worked its magic. Add to this the sounds of lapping water all around, the gondolas serenely paddling along the waterways, allowing us the time to simply 'be', and it really could not have been bettered. Walking the elegant pedestrian bridges, it felt as though we were on another planet.

The stunning, graceful beauty of the ancient stone buildings, and the lively music of Italian conversation, provided the tonic we so badly needed. We sauntered around the churches and galleries, people-watched as we sipped coffee and tea at cafés and enjoyed lingering meals together. It was perfect! We got royally lost, but who doesn't get lost in Venice? We panicked somewhat, then recovered and found our hotel – which was just as well, since we had forgotten its name.

On our last evening, as we ate, I took Miriam's hand. 'Thank you,' I said. 'For making all this happen. It's just the fairytale experience we needed.' Then, breathing in the fragrant air I said, 'It's allowed me to forget.'

'The dementia?'

I nodded. 'I don't think I've been capable of having a thought that wasn't about Alzheimer's in some way or other, not since the diagnosis. I'm sorry. Really I am, and I promise I'll try and manage it better.'

'You'd better,' she said. Then, lifting her glass, holding it out towards mine she said, '*Salute!*' And, clinking glasses, we toasted my resolution.

The journey home, however, shattered the idyll, bringing my new reality back to me at thundering speed. Stress was magnified for the once-simple tasks of preparing for a journey: packing, sorting tickets, catching the water bus to the mainland and the train to the airport. I fretted about being late, about losing paperwork or key codes. I fretted about losing my money. Fretting. Fretting. Worrying. 'Who is this new me?' I muttered to myself. 'And why is he taking over?'

And then there was the departure gate to negotiate: the queues to endure, the security to go through, the car to locate in Dublin. All of these small things that were once second nature to me had become a trial. Earlier in the summer I'd left my diary on a Ryanair flight and, although I'd

written to the airline asking for it back, I'd had no response.
That had rattled me, especially as it contained my thoughts
around the time of my diagnosis – memories I was unlikely
to be able to reclaim. But this time we managed the whole
journey with all my belongings intact.

I was congratulating myself about this as the car drew
into the drive and I took the bags into the house. It was
when I walked into my office that the trouble started. I
wanted to check my computer, to make sure that everything
was shipshape and ready for the working week. But where
was my computer? It wasn't in its habitual place on my desk.

'Miriam,' I said, 'have you seen my laptop?'

She popped her head out of the bedroom. 'Isn't it in
your office?'

'No,' I said. 'Obviously I've looked here. But it's disappeared.'

'Well, there's no sign of a break-in,' said Miriam. 'It
must be where you left it.'

At those words, 'break-in', I remembered. Before we'd
left, nervous that there would indeed be a burglary, I had
hidden my laptop. I remembered distinctly finding a good
place to hide it, but I couldn't recall where that place might
be. I shut my eyes in concentration, but it didn't help. I simply could not remember.

I sighed in frustration, and this was followed by anger
with myself, and then full-blown panic. In jig time I had
transformed the incident into a crisis. I *needed* the computer.
I needed it *now* to halt this overwhelming and unfamiliar
level of anxiety.

I rushed around, my heart racing, as I tore the house
apart, ransacking cupboards, reaching up to the highest

shelves, searching everywhere to no avail. Then I ran outside and stomped around the garden, fretting, my panic fuelled by the fact that I didn't recognise myself in this rampaging man.

Eventually I calmed myself down, steadied my breathing, walked the garden slowly and then, at last, the memory of where I had put the computer floated gently into my mind. It was behind a cushion in the sitting room. All had ended well, but it was a stark lesson. And it showed the narrowness of the gap between the controlled calm I showed the world, and the increasing vulnerability of my inner life.

By late autumn my professional life was proving highly stressful. The panto, *Peter Pan*, was gathering momentum, and there were the ongoing negotiations for the spring production of *I, Keano*. These had become a bruising and tiring chore.

As Line Manager of the panto I was responsible for streamlining the whole production process, which involved meeting the entire team. Year by year, the production was becoming increasingly ambitious, with more glitzy special effects like pyrotechnics. And although the production ran close to Christmas, we started planning early. The show was picked, and the tone decided on early in the year and, by early summer, the core team of seven would be hard at work. My job was to hold auditions, choose the cast, negotiate with the actors' agents, coordinate everything – the design, scenery and music – and make sure the production was running to budget.

In the past all this had been second nature to me. And as a result my reputation for being fair, decisive and good at my job meant that much was expected of me. Now I was terrified of making a mistake. I spent hours double-checking and triple-checking all the figures and details. I looked back with a sense of nostalgia at the days when I'd got a buzz out of all the multitasking. Now it was all about the preservation of my reputation and the maintenance of my income.

However, there was still satisfaction to be gained. But where, once, that came from achieving a near-impossible task and of getting my own way in the process, now my pleasure came more simply: I relished interacting with my colleagues. The knowledge that I was easing the journey for the production team pleased me greatly. It was enough.

When I watched the final rehearsals of *Peter Pan* in late November, I was impressed. The production seemed set for a successful run. But even while I sat there and basked in a vicarious glory – playing the politics of service – I was aware that the success of the production had little to do with my input. The director and choreographer, Daryn Crosbie, was the driver of all the ideas, I'd merely helped put them in place.

Early in December, John and Moya came to Miriam's annual felting exhibition. It was a bright, sunny day and, as I showed them round the house, with the light shining through the windows, and walked them down to the lake, it was looking its radiant best. They complimented me fulsomely.

'There was just a chalet here when we bought it,' I told them. 'And we couldn't have built this house without *Riverdance*.'

We talked of family, the fundamentals of living well and the trials that test us. It was wonderful to have such a positive exchange after weathering the often-complex politics of our working relationship.

Meanwhile, the panto season got into full swing. This was to be the last year in which I'd have to cope with the stresses alone – in the new year I would have an assistant and a trainee.

When earlier in the year I had told Caroline Desmond, Managing Director of The Gaiety Theatre, about my diagnosis, it wasn't yet common knowledge. Being supportive, Caroline was happy for me to stay on until I made the decision to retire, and I didn't plan on leaving for a while. But a week after my meeting with Caroline a knock came at my door. It was Leo McKenna, a young and keen junior Stage Manager on the pantomime.

'Hello Leo,' I said, beckoning him in. 'What can I do for you?'

I was expecting him to present me with a problem or perhaps with a complaint. So when he said rather bluntly, 'Ronan, can I have your job?' I was gobsmacked.

'No. *I've* got my job, thank you very much,' I said, feeling affronted.

'Oh.' He looked downcast. 'Is it not true, then?'

'Is what not true? What have you heard?' I asked, rather dreading the reply.

'That you're leaving?'

'Ah!'

I asked him where he'd heard this, and he said it was all around the theatre. He'd checked with his immediate boss, Daryn, before coming to see me. 'I asked him if he'd back me if I went for the position,' he said.

'And he agreed?'

He shrugged, and I got the impression Daryn's support had been somewhat half-hearted. Looking downcast, Leo turned for the door.

I liked Leo. I knew him well and respected him too. I'd met him first when we took the Abbey Theatre's production of *The Shadow of a Gunman* to Australia. At that time he was only fourteen and was accompanying his mother, the actress Bernadette McKenna, but he had impressed me with his maturity and ability to mix.

I'd employed him on *Riverdance* when he was in his early twenties. He was an ambitious young man and had already worked in the Gate Theatre for some years as a Stage Manager. Impressed with him, I put him on tour in the States. He worked well for the company and I had enjoyed my dealings with him, so I was surprised, and a little disappointed, when after less than two years with the company he had handed in his notice. Hadn't he seen what a great and unprecedented opportunity *Riverdance* was?

'I can't deal with the road life anymore,' he'd said. 'I know some people love it, but for me, having to go to my seventeenth hotel in three weeks? Well, no thanks!'

I thought over his proposition for a day or two and a plan started to form in my mind. I talked it over with Miriam. 'Leo is a good manager,' I said, 'and with his background he has a great understanding of theatre, but in my opinion he's not yet ready to make a success of the role of Line Manager. Not yet. But when I can no longer carry on, he'd be an ideal candidate to take over my job.'

'And you could train him up,' said Miriam, mirroring my idea. 'And he could undertake the tasks that you find difficult.'

'That's exactly what I was thinking,' I said. 'I could certainly do with some help. It's an arrangement that might suit us both.'

The following week, having consulted with Caroline and Daryn, I called him in. I told him of my diagnosis but explained that I had no intention of retiring anytime soon. Then I put my proposal to him.

'Leo, how would it be if you come in and work with me?' I said. 'You can help me out with some of the routine work, leaving me to concentrate on the day-to-day decisions and any problems that might ensue. And then, when I do leave, you will have the experience and expertise to have my job.'

We talked it over, and how this might work. And we began to plan. We agreed that Leo should keep on his job as Stage Manager for the current season – but that he could move across and work with me in 2015. Knowing that was in place took a weight off my shoulders. I could face the new year with a sense of ease.

Sixteen

Trying to Live Positively

The diagnosis, back in March 2014, had thrown up one particular anxiety. Could my brand of Alzheimer's be hereditary? Given that my father had suffered, and that I was diagnosed at a similar age, it seemed all too possible that this might be the case. After reading up the statistical likelihood, I asked to be tested.

As there are implications in this – in that if it did turn out to be hereditary there was a real possibility I would hand on the illness to my beautiful children, something impossible to contemplate – I was given genetic counselling before the doctors agreed that the test could be carried out. Then my samples and details wended their way to a high-tech laboratory in Switzerland for analysis.

I worried about the children. Hannah was twenty-two by now, and Loughlin nineteen. Complex ages where, starting out in life, they were crossing the bridge from childhood to young adults, a tricky terrain in the best of circumstances. How would they cope with the reality of my diagnosis?

I decided to be clear and real about my future, as I saw it. I explained that I could have a further fifteen years, even if no successful treatment could be found. By this time I was taking several drugs for the condition and, although they could alleviate my symptoms and hopefully slow my decline, they couldn't work a miracle. Hannah and Loughlin took this in calmly, but did, I noticed, adopt an attentive and practical watchfulness over me.

Around that time, in late autumn, a friend visiting our house brought with him his father who was well into the middle stages of dementia. He was calm and gentle, displaying no alarming signs. Hannah was at home at the time, and I noticed her watching him quietly. I imagined that she was projecting into the future, wondering how I would be in time.

I wanted more than anything to protect her and, feeling a sudden and overwhelming surge of anger against the condition, I left the room in order to calm myself. Stepping into my office, I told myself that predicting the future was a mug's game. 'I am not my father. I'm doing things he never did,' I said to myself, and listed those things. Exercise. Excellent diet. Mindfulness. Adequate rest. A good work-life balance. 'My journey is unknown,' I said out loud. Then, my calm restored, I returned to chat to our visitors.

In January, it was time to 'come out' to the wider public. And for the first time since 1989, when I had appeared on *The Late Late Show* with Gay Byrne, I found myself talking about my life with Alzheimer's. The first interview was for the health supplement of the *Irish Independent*. Deciding to adopt a 'can-do' stance, I reiterated the mantra I had formulated on the walk with Pepsi all those months ago. I stressed how in particular the Paleo Diet, which was devoid of refined sugar and cereal grain, had produced great health benefits for me.

Talking to the journalist Edel O'Connell, who was writing the piece, had been an odd experience in some ways.

The interview made me feel vulnerable yet excited, shy yet assertive. It was certainly different from the experience of talking about my father. Being the patient, and not the carer, made it uncomfortably close to the bone. I was captive, a person who was to slowly disappear.

I rather dreaded seeing what the journalist would make of me, but when the article was published on 9 January 2015, I was pleasantly surprised. The tone was measured and considered, and proved a true depiction of the points I had wanted to put across. I particularly liked the headline: 'Preparation, positivity and a Paleo diet helped me to cope with an Alzheimer's diagnosis at 56'. That said it all. It was a gentle easing back into advocacy.

Six weeks later I was asked to go on the RTÉ TV show *The Saturday Night Show*, presented by the journalist Brendan O'Connor. And while this was a bigger ordeal, it was equally a perfect opportunity to share my story and spread awareness.

I prepared nervously and was ready, only to be bumped off the show by a sixty-seven-year-old former Junior Minister who had come out as gay in order to support the Equal Marriage Rights constitutional referendum.

'We'd like you on next Saturday instead,' the researcher told me.

That gave me another week to agonise about the exposure and to worry about the egotism of the exercise. Of course it wasn't *about* me, not really; I was simply the conduit for the condition. Determined to get the salient points across so that the interview served its purpose in spreading awareness, I spent hours deliberating on what I was going to say. It was imperative that I decide the best points to focus on in order to aid people's understanding.

It felt strange, waiting nervously in the wings for the moment Brendan O'Connor would give the introduction. I heard him say, 'I'm going to play something for you now. This is a tape of an interview done back in the 1980s.' My own voice came on, talking to Gay Byrne about my father's Alzheimer's. Then he said, 'A year ago Ronan Smith was, himself, diagnosed with the same illness.'

As I stood up, ready to make my entrance, I heard the audience emit a loud, involuntary gasp of shock. It was like the sound of an audience at a Victorian melodrama. The empathy of that moment nearly unseated my focus. Was I crazy to be doing this?

I thought of Miriam who, along with Hannah and Loughlin, was sitting beside the audience, waiting. What would they make of this, and was it fair to put them through it? But, aware of the green light flashing above me, indicating that it really was time that I should enter, I marched onto the set.

As I sat down in the interview chair I could see my family, who were in my view, but out of the view of the cameras. Miriam sat between Hannah and Loughlin, they were all holding hands tightly.

With the audience clearly on my side, the interview went smoothly. I talked of my mantra – prepare, work, hope – and I was able to explain the need to keep healthy. Then, talking of the need for greater awareness, I said my hope was that people would overcome the awkwardness of encountering dementia. 'That's so important,' I said, 'for the sake of the sufferer as well as their carer.'

The rest went as I had, rather obsessively, planned. Brendan O'Connor was focused and keen, and the trade of a human-interest personal disclosure for a few minutes of mass-media public time was done.

It had been a performance, and I had kept to the script and delivered the goods.

Afterwards I was brought off stage by the floor manager and, with some relief, joined Miriam and the children in the green room. They all hugged me and said, 'Well done', and the researcher Ian assured me that the interview had gone well. 'It was extremely powerful,' he said. RTÉ had booked us into the Conrad Hotel, opposite the National Concert Hall, so we made our way there.

The next day Julian Erskine and his wife Anita Reeves invited all four of us over for brunch. 'Then we can all watch *The Saturday Night Show* together,' Anita had said when she issued the invitation.

As we drove there, having breakfasted well at the hotel, Miriam mentioned what a great kindness this was.

'Kindness? But Miriam, they're our friends,' I said, not understanding what she meant.

'It's an acknowledgment,' she said, 'that they understand what we're all going through. They sense that it would be difficult for us to just go home, watch as a family and carry on as normal. They're giving us time to pause and mull everything over. It's like they're saying, "You're going through this ordeal. We understand it's hard. We're inviting you into our lives with your lives."'

When we arrived and were welcomed in, swept up and presented with a quite beautiful brunch, I began to understand what Miriam meant. We chatted about the theatre, about *Riverdance*, and Julian told a few anecdotes about our time working together, which greatly amused the children.

Then they turned on the TV, set the recorder and we sat down to watch the show.

I wasn't sure how it would affect me, watching back, but I viewed it all quite dispassionately. I think it was harder for the children watching again, seeing it on TV.

Anita was visibly moved by the interview, moved and I think a little shocked. I felt the reality of her reaction, and afterwards she gave us space to talk and voice all our worries and the uncertainties of the future. This willingness to listen – and to let the whole family be real with her and Julian – meant a lot to me, but perhaps even more to Miriam. 'I feel there's a scaffold of support around us,' she said as we drove home.

For the following few days, messages of congratulation poured in. That was gratifying. And then, predictably, the glory faded as the world moved on and I was left with the memories the media frenzy had stirred up.

Now that my worries over publicity were behind me, I had to address the weightier concerns about my work. A crisis had reared its head in *I, Keano* land. Our leading man fell sick and dropped out just a week before rehearsals were due to start, and I had yet to find a PR-friendly celebrity to make up the cast. This was all a little too enervating for me in my current super-stressed state.

The situation sorted itself out, as these things are wont to do, and the first reading rehearsal took place. It went well. As I sat in the company of excited actors, the air crackled with waves of energy, bonhomie and optimism. Falling in with the mood, nostalgia swept me back to my acting days and a wave of sadness washed over me.

Spring saw my mood take a further dip. I was part of a downbeat panel discussion after a showing of *Still Alice*, a depressing, and rather Hollywood depiction of how Alzheimer's can progress, in this case showing a university professor's alarmingly fast decline. And if that wasn't enough to dent my mood, the death of Terry Pratchett at sixty-six – just eight years after he contracted the disease – really drove the message home.

However much you work at prevention – at watching your diet, keeping your brain active and balancing your life, it's difficult to remain optimistic and believe that you might beat the disease when the world is showing you a more pessimistic view.

I voiced all this to Miriam.

'That doesn't mean that you'll only have eight years,' she said, noticing how morose I had become after this double dose of gloom.

'It's the average timeline,' I said.

'But neither Terry Pratchett nor you is average,' said Miriam. 'Nobody is. That's what you keep telling me. Every case is unique.'

I'm lucky, I told myself later in the month as I walked along the side of the lake, the spring sunshine setting in rose-coloured hues on the still water. Watching Pepsi scampering ahead, tail wagging in constant motion, I felt restful and at ease. For a second or two. But then the twinge of bitter anticipated loss rolled in. Sighing, I thought, 'Even the beauty of nature is compromised by the fatalism that now haunts me.'

Life became a constant game of hunt the thimble, or more accurately hunt the glasses, hunt the keys, the diary or the mobile phone. Or the fountain pen I am so very fond of. It was like a rolling loss and recovery programme:

at any one time, at least one of these things would be absent. I was constantly having to trawl through my brain and retrace my steps to find where the object had been put down and abandoned.

This interrupted my days and it irked me considerably. But over time I came to accept it as part of my new life, still irritating, yes, but as natural to me now as breathing. Less easy to accept was my constant fretting over each small task.

By now the rehearsals for *I, Keano* were in full swing and the fifteen-to sixteen-hour days left me bone tired. The production was excellent and the audience enthusiastic, but the bookings were low and, sadly, with its projected cost of half a million euros, it could only be considered a failing enterprise.

My next project was for the Alzheimer Society of Ireland (ASI). They asked me to take part in a seminar in the Long Room Hub in Trinity College Dublin: I was to give a first-person perspective examining the stigma associated with the condition. I agreed, seeing this as a great opportunity to help the cause, but was a little anxious of speaking in front of an audience of eighty, made up of carers, medical professionals, journalists and students.

I stood up, determined to deliver my message with strong conviction. I started well, and was beginning to believe that I had achieved this aim. As I was nearing the end, however, and was speaking of the Alzheimer's sufferer's human right to dignity and respect – even and perhaps especially during the final decline – my voice cracked. A wave of emotion washed over me. Annoyed with myself, I felt my speech had come across as a desperate plea rather than the firm demand I had intended.

The following week saw me participating in a workshop at the Irish Museum of Modern Art. They were exploring the potential for conducting tours for those with dementia and, given my diagnosis coupled with my history in the arts, asked for my contribution.

Offering a suggestion, I began to describe how dementia had affected my life. I gave a dispassionate view and, when I glanced up, noticed one participant well up with tears. It struck me then that coping with this thing day-to-day makes me forget how bloody sad the condition is. Emotion is never far from the surface when dementia is present. It strikes at the very heart of humanity.

This was on my mind when, days later, I walked from our house up Pound Lane to a small monument on Black Hill, where a British plane had crashed in heavy fog returning from a bombing raid on Germany during World War II. It's a place that always provokes melancholy and, plodding on stubbornly against the unseasonal gusts of strong wind, I tried to assess my mood objectively. And I concluded that when my brain wasn't preoccupied with work, family or social engagements, it tended to slip into sadness. Was that now my destiny?

Then I reflected on my decline, and on the deterioration of my functions. How would I react in the future? Would I accept my decline and be benign, easy in myself and in the way I related to my carers? This thought led to one tantalising question. To what degree could I exercise choice in how I handled it? Could I choose equanimity? Could I control my response? I would certainly try.

At this stage, my diagnosis was still 'probable early-onset Alzheimer's', but as the summer went on I had accumulated enough evidence of struggle and dysfunction to recognise that the word 'probable' could now be discounted. I was suffering the pathology of a progressive, if oh so slowly progressive, neurological disorder.

And when I attended my second genetic counselling appointment with Miriam by my side, the diagnosis was clear. The result was positive. No sooner had I scratched the word 'probable' from my mind, the doctor delivered yet another hammer blow. A mutation had been found in the PSEN gene, which meant my Alzheimer's was genetic. I could stop wondering how I had 'caught' it; *it* had caught *me*!

As I sat there absorbing my new reality, the doctor told me that the inherited form is very rare. 'Recent research statistics rate it as somewhere around one per cent of the global dementia population,' he said, explaining that the remaining ninety-nine per cent of patients have sporadic Alzheimer's disease, which has no known cause.

'You mean I'm part of an exclusive club?' I quipped, trying to spike some humour into this grim consultation.

'Well yes, though not, I would imagine, one you were keen to join,' he said with a wry smile. He then reeled off a number of names and acronyms for my condition. It can be called Familial Alzheimer's Disease (FAD), or sometimes Dominantly Inherited Alzheimer's Disease (DIAD). He also mentioned that trials were underway, called Dominantly Inherited Network Trials Unit (DIAN-TU). Miriam carefully wrote them all down.

'They don't make it easy, do they?' she muttered, reading through her notes as we made our way home.

I laughed. 'I think they might make up these kinds of acronyms so that we patients get some cognitive exercise.'

'In remembering them, you mean?' said Miriam with an answering chuckle. 'Perhaps you're right.'

Although it seemed easier to make light of it all, in truth, the latest diagnosis hadn't hit me very hard. If I felt anything about this new piece of news, it was a sense of numbness. In essence, nothing had changed. I still had the disease, whatever the cause. I was still having to fight the progression of it, while hoping against hope for some timely, effective treatment. This wouldn't change the way I chose to live.

It wasn't until later that evening, letting Pepsi out and noticing a sky full of stars, that reality suddenly hit. If this was a genetic form of Alzheimer's, there was a chance that I would pass it on to my beautiful children. It was simply too terrible to contemplate. The realisation had raked the coals of useless anger into life again. And as always in my worst moments, my thoughts turned to my father, and how his anger had eventually abated. And how, at the end, his presence was an absence. What had that felt like? Had he suffered? Would I?

Around this time I got a chance to remember my father in his glory days. One of his proudest moments had been hearing his own Brendan Smith Theatre Academy referred to as 'Ireland's RADA' (Royal Academy of Dramatic Art) in the British press. Of all his lifetime achievements, the school was the one closest to his heart. The business was entirely his, he had no partners, no investors and no funds from government agencies.

When The Lir Academy, a full-time, third-level per-forming arts school, opened in Dublin – a school which was linked to RADA – I thought it would be appropriate for my father's portrait to hang there. Painted by Robert Ballagh, the portrait was currently hanging in the Olympia Theatre, but the move was duly agreed to and carried out.

It wasn't long before Miriam and I discussed the possibility of the children inheriting this beastly disease. Should we tell them? Well, obviously they would have to know, but first I wanted to arm myself with all the available information. There wasn't much, and what there was didn't give me much cause for optimism.

If a parent carries the mutated gene then, based on present global statistics, there is a fifty per cent possibility of the mutated gene being transmitted on each and every separate conception. So basically the toss of a coin: heads, you will get the illness, tails you won't. And there was nothing, absolutely nothing that I could do to change any of this. What would this information do for my children? What would they do with it?

Both children have lived away from home since they started college, so we waited until they visited at the weekend to present them with the news. In the event, Hannah and Loughlin shrugged it off, concentrating only on what this firm diagnosis meant for me. They both declined testing, saying there were years to go before they had to worry, by which time there would probably be a cure. 'We want to concentrate on you,' said Hannah. 'That's all that matters to us.'

Life continued on its rocky, rollercoaster way. One minute I was positive, enthusiastically following my dietary and exercise regimes; the next, my mood blackened. When that happened it felt as if I'd been mugged. All my strategies withered and collapsed like a sadly deflated balloon, and I was left with nothing but deep hurt. It took immense effort to pull myself back, but I blinked hard, shook my head and marshalled my thoughts. And went back to 'fighting the good fight' one more time.

In late October 2015 I was busy working on preparations for the panto, *Little Red Riding Hood*, at The Gaiety. My side-kick Leo had proved a delight to work with: he was a willing student, he accepted my mentoring and we had an excellent working relationship. Now that the pace was building with rehearsals due to start, I was especially grateful for his help.

Leo and I differed in many ways. I am extremely – some would say obsessively – tidy, and kept all my papers neatly in filing cabinets, whereas Leo liked to use the entire office floor; but rather than rankling, that was just a cause for amusement between us. We worked happily together and in harmony.

I was also hard at work with the ASI. I did a series of talks on the living experience at events and conferences, and at each one I became more proficient. As I became more resigned to the realities of the condition, the sudden rush of emotions that had hijacked my talks in the past started to dissipate. I was growing in confidence and more able to con-tribute in a useful and hopefully beneficial way. Following on from pioneer speakers like Helen Rochford Brennan and Kathy Ryan, fellow sufferers of the disease, talks like these were a significant factor in helping to remove any stigma and encourage better understanding and openness.

As I spoke at the third event of a series of three, this time for the Irish Hospice Association, I enthusiastically shared the mantra I had devised, and even as the words describing 'the need to work for the possible' were leaving my mouth, I realised with a certain disconsolateness that I had failed to follow through on my own advice. 'This,' I thought wryly, 'was a classic case of physician, heal thyself!'

I had made a start though, to be fair. I'd initiated the various legal steps required to set things up for the family but had not followed them through to completion. I had tried the art of meditation but had not put in place a sustained practice.

Some months earlier, Miriam had booked us into a weekend at a Buddhist retreat, and we'd joined a group of twenty for a series of guided meditations. On Saturday the priest said we were to have a silent meditation for the evening, keeping up the silence while we prepared and ate dinner. This was challenging, but I tried my very best, and I thought I'd managed okay.

But when the group assembled for a wind-down session on Sunday before we left, I mentioned my diagnosis of Alzheimer's and the group burst into gales of laughter. 'So that's why you kept talking,' they said. I joined in the merriment but have to admit I hadn't thought I'd broken the silence too noticeably often. I mentioned this to Miriam on the way home and laughing, she said, 'Ronan, you kept talking! Everyone was asking you to shush.'

I went home from the conference with a new determination. I would pay proper attention to my own advice while I still had the capacity to do so. Time was of the essence.

But how could I prepare for the loss of my mind? How could I be sure that all the strategies and plans I was currently devising could possibly be maintained? It's a terrible thing having to surrender part of oneself. I've never much liked the notion of Alzheimer's as 'a living death' as it seems reductionist and melodramatic, but it does, I fear, capture the guts of the thing.

I was feeling distinctly sorry for myself when an interview with John Hume's wife was aired on the radio. She was talking about being his carer through his dementia and was recounting, with great simplicity and honesty, the bitter sadness of living with the person you loved, but having to answer the same question twenty times a day. She emphasised the patience it demands along with the hurt it generates.

Listening, my sadness redirected itself towards Miriam. If the Beast gives such symptoms to me, as I assumed he will, I will then inflict this pain on her. How can I do that? And how to hold on to any kind of hope? My thoughts turned black. All the huff and puff of positivity, the fight-back advocacy, the public speaking seemed hopeless in the face of the persistence of this cruel, relentless progression.

I had seen a great deal of my old friend Philip Lee during 2015. He and Una visited us at home, we'd dined with them, and he and I had met on a regular basis in order to catch up with each other's lives. He was, without fail, a good friend and support to me.

I had of course discussed my dilemma with him, and my thoughts on how I could cope with the thought of losing my mind, and he suggested I meet with Ian Robertson, Professor of Psychology at Trinity College Dublin. In fact, he did more, and made an introduction. It was a useful meeting. Many of Robertson's observations resonated with me, but the main message I brought home was one of hope.

'Ronan, you're an example of a new kind of Alzheimer's patient,' he said. 'By using regimes of physical exercise, conscious cognitive exercise, diet and a positive mindset, you don't fit into the existing statistics. You're an experiment. Who knows how it's going to work out?'

His words were the best of Christmas presents. I faced into the festive season with a real sense of hope and good cheer.

Seventeen

The Final Curtain

The cheer of welcoming in 2016 was somewhat dented in January, when I took a cognitive test. This was part of a drug trial programme that I had started a number of months earlier. By this stage in my illness, the form of these tests was familiar to me and, as I did them, I was horribly aware that I was not performing as well as I had the last time.

I didn't think the change was dramatic – it was perhaps marginal – but it charted a real progression, slight but certain. This dose of reality left me with a wave of resentment.

I was mulling it over the following day when I set off in the car to deliver a parcel to neighbours. The address, Three Castles, is a bare kilometre or two away from home. It's a place I know like the back of my hand, as it's on a cycle route that I regularly use. Why then was I circling the roads with no idea of where, exactly, the house was?

I pulled up at the side of the road and tried to gather my thoughts. I could see the house in my mind's eye, but I couldn't link that information with its exact location. And in that rural place, there were no street names to put me back on course. I sat there and panicked.

It took twenty minutes before I managed to reorient myself. Twenty minutes of driving around randomly.

But even when I found the house, I couldn't work out how I had got lost, nor how I had eventually found my way. It was hard to admit it, but I saw it for what it was. Dysfunction and degeneration, pure and simple. My mind was in turmoil as I drove home. With my shrinking capacity came the diminishing of my world. I was losing my identity, and this put me in a rolling state of grief.

I was busy with meetings, rushing from Alzheimer's advocacy meetings to panto talks in The Gaiety. They jostled against each other like clumsy bedfellows. After the final performance of *Little Red Riding Hood* one the stars, Nick Grennell, came over and thanked me. Saying how much he always enjoyed the gig, in spite of the long hours and gruelling work, he added that much of that was down to me. 'You look after us so well, Ronan,' he said, 'and much of the success of the production comes from your calm and supportive supervision.'

It was nice to hear that I hadn't lost my touch. And it reinforced my decision to continue to remain as the people person, the one the team came to with its problems. That was something I could do and was good at.

In February, when I chaired the pantomime production team post-mortem, there was a productive and positive working atmosphere. That was good. But after the stress I'd encountered over the run of the panto, I decided to hand over more of the logistics to Leo.

It was a win-win situation: good and right for me, for Leo and for the theatre. Since the illness would inevitably progress, forcing me to delegate, how much better it was to anticipate this and take action beforehand. Had I ploughed on regardless, the production inevitably would have suffered and, mimicking my father before me, I would have become a liability. For all that, this move came with sadness.

I had been invited to join a Health Service Executive Committee working on a public information campaign. I attended the 'Understand Together' meetings enthusiastically enough, but can't claim that the other committee members always liked what I had to say.

At one of the meetings someone said that there should never be an air of depression around the diagnosis. I gave a knee-jerk reaction. 'Well it *is* depressing news,' I said. 'There's really no up-side, is there? It's just a challenge to cope with.'

There was an awkward silence around the table. Nobody dared to argue with the person with dementia, it seemed. There was a polite chorus of throat clearing, then the meeting moved on.

The truth was that my dysfunction was increasing. What I did yesterday disappeared into a fog that took an applied and focused effort to dispel. There was a slow and plodding process of retrieval. If someone said, 'I'll see you at three at the square in Rathdrum', it took me time and energy to work out where Rathdrum was.

Deciding to formalise my path towards retirement, I spoke to my boss Caroline Desmond in May. I asked for a fee increase and said I'd like to work for two more years as Line Producer, assisted by Leo McKenna, and then revert to being a Consultant Producer after that. We shook on the deal.

All these plans for the ending of my career had me thinking about the start of it. And when in June I attended the unveiling of a portrait of playwright Bernard Farrell at the Abbey Theatre, I met a crowd of old friends and was reminded of those early years, those halcyon days when I secured great parts and seemed to be at the start of a promising acting career. Those memories of thirty years ago came flooding back with an echo of the excitement that had accompanied my young adult life.

Contemplating this I wondered if, over the past twenty years, I had been hiding my true self. In following the path of middle-class pragmatist careerist, had I had mere pretensions of creativity? Had I bottled my dreams?

There were cheery events to punctuate the everyday trials of daily life. Thanks to Philip I'd joined a group of cyclists that would meet at weekends for breakfast before cycling in the Wicklow hills.

Julian Erskine took up kayaking. Becoming keener, he bought a second, better kayak, and brought them both over to Lacken some weekends. We loved this, and when Miriam suggested we should get a double kayak so that all three of us could enjoy the lake together, I agreed at once.

I often lunched with Julian in my days working at The Gaiety, and one afternoon he brought me to the Great Outdoors shop where we picked out an excellent double kayak. We go out frequently. Being *on* the lake – on the water I generally look out on, has proved a wonderfully calming experience. It has become a great solace in our lives. How lucky I am in my friends and where I live!

We celebrated our twenty-sixth wedding anniversary quietly with the children, Hannah's partner James, and Loughlin's girlfriend Eve. Enjoying their easy company,

I thanked my lucky stars, and Miriam, that we had such a close and reassuringly warm family.

The summer of 2016 saw a noticeable change in my capabilities, or at least in my reaction to them. Miriam and I were planning a trip to India, in a group with friends, something we were both looking forward to. First, I had to sort out the visas – simple enough you would think. But it was somewhat convoluted, and the very thought of negotiating the twists and turns of multiple visits to the Indian Embassy sent my stress levels into orbit. And if that worried me, how on earth would I manage the trip?

As it turned out, we never did go to India. Miriam, who had been so looking forward to this break away, was unlucky enough to suffer a break of another kind. Just three days before our departure date she fell in the garden and broke her leg. She was stoic, as she always is, but I could sense her devastation.

My disappointment, however, was tinged with relief. My obsession with my illness had reached greater depths. It was affecting my social life too: by now the thought of keeping up with the conversation in a group was more of a challenge than a pleasure.

At dinner parties and gatherings I started tuning out of friends' conversations. All I wanted to talk about was my health. To voice the thing that consumed so much of my thinking. But I dreaded becoming a dementia bore. I'd rap myself on the knuckles, and tell myself, 'Down boy! Get back into your cage!'

In July I fell victim to an internet scam. The sum wasn't too significant – I lost five hundred euro – but the humiliation flattened me. Deeply ashamed of being taken in, I kept the incident to myself. But it reminded me starkly of the time my father, lost in Paris, suffered an admittedly more serious scam. Like father, like son.

Miriam had organised a surprise for Hannah's twenty-third birthday. She had made complicated plans, scheduling events at a series of locations.

'Don't you dare blow it all,' she warned me, taking me through the logistics of the day.

She needn't have worried. On the day, I'd forgotten what the plans were, and had as much of a mystery tour as the birthday girl herself.

Sitting in the back of the car as Miriam and Hannah chatted happily in the front, I realised I was grieving. Grieving the loss of function, of potential. My world was closing, shrinking, diminishing. I'd lost my identity. I was now the man with Alzheimer's.

As my deterioration continued, so did Miriam's worries.

'How will I manage the tax affairs?' she said, watching me one day in the office. 'And the bill paying, the house maintenance, the repairs?'

I reassured her, saying there were experts she could employ who would manage that for her. 'And the children will help, I'm sure of that,' I said. 'And friends too. You know how much they long to be of use, to do something.'

Fortunately, we seemed to alternate, one of us being strong when the other was wobbly. We were an effective double act. And talking of those, I was coming up to my last double-plate-spinning professional work in the autumn of 2016. I'd thought the contained piece of work I'd recently taken on, helping out Barnstorm Theatre in Kilkenny, would be manageable, and although I did indeed manage it, the stress involved stepped out of the zone of healthy cognitive challenge into decidedly negative territory.

Clearing my head as I walked the beach with Pepsi, I realised my double-jobbing days were over. I was tired of the struggle. Listening to the small and gentle waves curling and collapsing on the shore wave after wave, I heard them as a steady and insistent message of exhaustion that matched my mood, then pulled it down further. To try and pull myself back I developed a new mantra. It was simple, or simple to say, if less so to employ. It was 'keep fighting, keep hoping, keep going'.

At this point the pattern broke and Miriam's mood matched mine. I had been her rock, but that rock, having become brittle, was now slowly crumbling. We were like battle-weary soldiers, each leaning on the other. 'This is hopeless,' she said one evening, as we both voiced our fears for the future. 'We'll have to adjust our tactics.'

Drinking our wine as we sat on a bench in her 'special garden', up high like the stage of a theatre, looking over the lake in the last of the September sunshine, we vowed to stop catastrophising about the future. 'Remember,' she said, 'we'll be positive, and active, and we'll live in the moment.'

I nodded. At least that would make the journey as supported and as comfortable as it could be for us both.

These new tactics were all very well, but back in the summer I had committed to giving a filmed talk, in the form of a TED Talk, on living with dementia. I'd have to present this to a live audience on behalf of the ASI. Planning it I promised Miriam, and myself, that this would be the last high hurdle of commitment I would jump over.

I prepared my talk with care, but had the greatest difficulty remembering what to say. I was in despair, but on that October evening as I drove into the Sugar Club in Dublin, I delivered a focused and fluid address to the windscreen while I was driving. There was to be live music interspersed between the talks. My pantomime colleagues had helped in this, they performed song and dance numbers. These additions proved inspirational, lifting the mood and creating a lively and engaged response to the talks. Mine went well! For the final dance, most of us – speakers, friends, carers and supporters – took to the stage to join the performers from The Gaiety in an uplifting dance.

'This is great,' Miriam said as we bopped around on the stage. And she was right! We were dancing for joy, and that encapsulated the best meaning of living with dementia. If only it could always be so.

As part of my preparation for retirement, I had been meeting with Geoff, my financial advisor. And now, for the first time, I took along two trusted friends. I'd deemed this necessary because of my rising trajectory of symptoms and, although it was unnerving to relinquish control and rely on the judgement of others, it turned out to have been a wise and necessary move.

It didn't take long for the conversation to outpace me, but instead of allowing myself to panic and give in to stress, I sat back quietly and let them get on with it. Sometimes it is best to let go.

Back at work, I forgot the notes I needed for a meeting in Kilkenny and had to ask Hannah to scan them and email them over to me. At The Gaiety, budgetary problems raised their head, not my fault (someone had overspent on props), but I felt the weight of responsibility.

When the principals were joined by the rest of the cast, the panto rehearsals started in earnest. The machine ground into life. Tasks began to accumulate, and each one took longer than was the case a year before. Much longer. It wasn't noticeable to others; I could fool them, but the Beast and I knew the truth of it.

Things were changing. There was the appearance and there was the reality. I appeared to be a Line Producer with a Line Producer-in-waiting by my side, but in reality Leo was already performing many functions of the role. And just as well too. I decided to take a back seat in 2017 and to retire at the end of that season, at sixty, rather than waiting for another year until 2018 as originally planned.

Nobody had questioned my ability to remain as Line Producer, no one had suggested it was time to leave. On the contrary, my colleagues made it very clear that my work was still valued. If I had been in any doubt of that – and there were inevitably times that I worried about it – watching that year's panto, *Robin Hood*, at one of the final rehearsals made all the work feel worthwhile. Caroline Desmond and I were crying with laughter. 'Daryn has done it again!' I said to her. 'We are so lucky to have him.'

She agreed and added, 'And we're lucky to have you! I know how much work you put in, Ronan. And I appreciate it.'

I arrived home that day in an ebullient mood to find Miriam equally buoyant. Her annual exhibition of her felting art had been well attended and sales had been high. Truly a double cause for celebration.

After some technical hitches, *Robin Hood* opened to widespread acclaim. I was happy and not a little bit relieved. The year had gone well, with the gradual handover to Leo, and I was now ready to approach Caroline with a new proposal.

It was this: I would be a Consulting Producer with no significant logistic or delivery responsibilities. I'd effectively be a strategy consultant and would be available to sort out all and any issues. This would apply through both the production and the run periods.

She agreed. And with the relief that followed came the inevitable sadness.

In December I was approached and asked to appear in a television documentary about Alzheimer's. The filming would take place at home and Miriam and the children would also appear. We talked this over and agreed that we would do it. And when on 10 December the cameras came in, we all played our parts.

With my workload lifted, I now cycled more regularly. When I mentioned this, the director asked if they could film me on my bike. I duly cycled up and down the road, first rehearsing the clip, then being filmed in a number of takes.

An hour later a phone call interrupted our lunch break. Miriam took the call and, after chatting a while, doubled over in laughter. Switching the phone off, she said it was Maria, a good friend and neighbour. 'She rang to see were you all right, Ronan. She'd seen you cycle up and down the road and thought you must be lost.'

'You mean that I'd lost it. That I'd forgotten where I live?'

'Exactly.'

The whole crew had a good laugh about that one.

Around the time *My Broken Brain* aired, there were a number of radio interviews and newspaper articles. I'm used

to that now. There were congratulatory calls, but the programme hadn't made a big media splash, it certainly hadn't
gone viral, and this disappointed me. I would love it if my
work with ASI made a real difference, if it truly spread
awareness and understanding.

Walking Pepsi, my mood a little low, I thought about
grieving and wondered if it's possible to grieve for the loss
of yourself without descending into self-pity. It's never considered self-pity if you're grieving for someone else, and how
can something be about yourself yet of yourself? It was a
riddle, and I was trying to understand it.

My short-term memory was becoming increasingly
compromised. Writing my diary, I found myself scratching
my head to work out what I had done the day before. It took
minutes of dredging to remember I'd attended a neighbour's
child's birthday tea. Yet I had enjoyed the afternoon, and
had chatted away amiably.

While it was good having no pressure of day-to-day
work, I did find that time hung heavy. There was much to
be done around the house and garden, and much paperwork to trawl through, but I didn't feel inclined to get
through the to-do list. Besides, it took a lot of checking
and worry to find out just what was on that list of four or
five items.

I had, however, begun to write. After years of procrasti-
nation, I had finally started real work on a book I'd planned:
a memoir of my father's Alzheimer's journey, and my own.
I'd made a start in 2015, but barely managed five minutes
at a time. I was now in a good routine. I was writing for a
solid two hours each day and making substantial progress.
That was gratifying.

The close of 2017 was bittersweet. I ploughed on, managing my last panto, *Rapunzel*, enjoying my new role, able to mostly hide any cognitive or memory struggles from my colleagues.

Caroline Desmond asked me how I felt about stepping down. 'You don't have to retire, Ronan,' she said. 'We'll be very happy for you to stay on if you want to.'

Thanking her, I explained that the stress any work engendered was becoming unhealthy, and she nodded her sympathy.

'You've made up your mind?'

I nodded. 'Yes,' I said. 'I have.'

'We'll be very sorry to lose you,' she said, mentioning, flatteringly, the value I brought to the panto. 'We all will. You've been such a support to all of us, and your negotiation skills are second to none.' Looking up, smiling, she said, 'What will we do without you!'

I could perhaps have stretched my final exit, but I wanted to manage my departure calmly and discreetly, without trauma.

Quite why, when my professional dilemmas were fixed, I should sink into the abyss again I don't know. But no positivism could counter the drudge of hauling myself into tasks that took a ridiculously long time to complete. The Beast had me well and truly on the run, it was closing in on me slowly and stealthily.

I tried so hard to live up to all that I was learning from, and contributing to, with the ASI. As a good advocate, it was important that I should show how to live well with dementia, something that crucially involves adapting to a deteriorating condition. It was about facing it, adjusting situations and surrendering things. It meant being real and honest about my decline.

Then two events happened that made me appreciate all that life had given me. First, Miriam organised a sixtieth birthday party, held a little before the day itself, in Tinakilly House near Wicklow. Seeing my wonderful family and loyal friends gathered together, hearing the eulogistic speeches, having Hannah and Loughlin sing to me and then, as the icing on the cake, having a private performance of *Riverdance* gifted by John and Moya – how could I not feel like the luckiest man alive? For that night at least.

And then there was the opening night of *Rapunzel*. First nights are a grand affair at The Gaiety. There were always invited guests, most of them from the world of showbiz. And there was a buzz of excitement as Miriam, Hannah and I made our way to our seats in the front row of the dress circle. Loughlin was in Barcelona at the time, at college there.

Looking around the theatre I spotted the TV and radio host Pat Kenny with his wife and children. Caroline Desmond smiled and waved from the Director's box as we all waited for the show to begin. It promised to be a good pantomime this year, if the rehearsals were anything to go by. Along with the stalwarts, Joe Conlan as the dame (nanny Ninny Noonah) and Nicholas Grennell as the king, we had some newcomers. Ciara Lyons, playing a teenager, promised to hold the stage with ease.

For some years Hannah had been my accomplice in some of this. In her early teenage years she had attended some pantomime rehearsals with me and, as she got older, she sat in on the auditions too. I'd ask her advice, and she showed an innate talent for casting. Later, I'd show her the script, inviting her to suggest improvements. She showed real insight. It was a wonderfully bonding father-daughter thing to do, and was very much our Saturday thing.

Hannah was interested in pursuing a management or production role in theatre. She had worked with Julian Erskine on *I, Keano*, as work experience during Transition Year at school. And now, having graduated from college, she had taken a series of theatre jobs.

It was one the most interactive pantos for years, and the audience positively lapped it up. The boos, the cheers, the 'Oh yes he is' and 'Oh no he isn't', all made for a fun performance. I wasn't surprised by the standing ovation, but I was pleased that the applause went on, seemingly forever. Sales had already been healthy and I suspected that, with this pantomime, an extension well into January was on the cards.

When the clapping finally ceased we reached for our coats, ready to make our way to the bar for our first-night drinks and nibbles. But Joe Conlan, standing at the edge of the stage, said, 'I have a special announcement to make.' Miriam caught my eye, questioningly, and I shrugged. There hadn't been any announcement in the script. And his next words staggered me.

'Our wonderful producer, Ronan Smith, is retiring soon, and today just happens to be his birthday.'

I groaned and felt like hiding. 'Could you all please turn your backs on the stage and look up at the dress circle?' A spotlight shone on my head. Blinking, I waved in acknowledgment. Then 'Happy Birthday' struck up and everyone – the cast, the crew and the audience – raised their voices and belted it out. It was so unexpected, so meaningful, that I felt a tear in my eye.

'That was wonderful,' said Miriam as, around us, friends and strangers alike smiled and added their wishes.

'Did you know?'

'Not a clue,' she said. 'What a pity Loughlin isn't here.'

When we walked into the bar I did a double take. The place was festooned with balloons and with banners saying 'Happy Birthday'. And not only that: where, in general, nibbles would be laid out on tables at first nights, now there were tables laid with linen tablecloths. Alan McQuillan, the Theatre Manager, approached us and led us to the head table. And there was my brother Julian and his wife.

The food was beautiful. When we had finished eating Caroline stood up to speak. I blushed at her words of praise and the reactions of all my colleagues, who intoned 'Hear, hear' at each of her flattering pronouncements.

After everyone had raised their glasses in a toast the lights dimmed and this enormous cake appeared, wheeled in on a trolley. There was an audible gasp as everyone took in the scene it depicted. The Gaiety stage had been replicated in icing and all these different, colourful characters were on the stage, performing. And in front of them, script in hand, was a bald-headed man.

'Wow,' said Hannah. 'Dad, that's you to a tee.'

More speeches followed: each, it seemed, more fulsome than the last. I watched Hannah's face as she listened, her pride and love clear to see. And I basked in her emotion. She and Miriam voiced their pride to me as we left the theatre. 'What an evening,' said Hannah. 'Dad, I'll remember that for the rest of my life.'

I smiled, happy. I wished I could say the same. That I too would remember it. But that simply would not have been true.

Eighteen

It's a Wrap

The new year of 2018 brought with it an unexpected problem. It was the end of January and I was driving home from town, slowly and carefully, in fairly heavy traffic. I drove up a winding road towards Blessington, and the next thing I knew I was waking from a strange dream to strangers who were peering in at me, asking if I was all right.

I squinted, trying hard to see, then slowly my vision cleared and my brain caught up with the fact that this was no dream – it was very real indeed. Still in my car, I was upside-down, in the ditch.

'Are you all right?' a man asked.

'I think so,' I said, still feeling a sense of unreality.

'Can you move your fingers? Your toes?'

I tried. 'Yes,' I said. 'All in working order.'

At that, the door opened, and I was helped out of my upside-down car.

'What happened?' I asked.

'The car just left the road. It crossed over, hit the kerb at an awkward angle and flipped. Do you not remember any of that?'

I shook my head. Part of me was still wondering if this *could* be a dream. But as the minutes passed, and an ambulance arrived to cart me off to accident and emergency, I had to accept, rather ruefully, that this was all too real.

I was lucky. I hadn't hit anyone, and the traffic around me had stopped immediately and safely. I spent several hours in accident and emergency; all my functions seemed intact. And I was questioned fully about all I could, and could not, remember.

'It seems you had a blackout,' said the doctor, jotting something down in a chart. 'I'd estimate that you were unconscious for five or six minutes.'

That bothered me. Miriam and I talked over the significance of this as she drove me home. But, recovering, I suffered no residual problems, and we let the matter lie for a while. But in March, travelling on the LUAS tram into town, I felt woozy and faint. After sitting still for several minutes I tentatively carried on with my day, but the feeling travelled with me. It was like a fog between me and the world. Could this be linked to the blackout? I told Miriam of this new development.

'Why don't we contact Des O'Neill?' she said, referring to one of Ireland's leading gerontologists.

'That's a good idea.' Des and I are friends, and our friendship goes back a long way. I'd met him at sixteen when the two of us were selected as part of a theatre group to go to Brussels to perform Wilde's *The Importance of Being Earnest*, and we'd kept in touch over the years. I had told him about my diagnosis and he promised to do all he could for me. 'Pick up the phone anytime,' he'd said, and now we took him at his word. He has played such a pivotal role in my life with Alzheimer's and is always there for me.

It was straight into Tallaght Hospital for me, where they ran various tests. Then I went to St James's syncope clinic to discover if the problem was linked to a tendency to faint. It wasn't. They ran a CT scan of my brain and, when that proved satisfactory, Des said that it might be my heart. He sent me to cardiologist David Moore, and I wore a loop monitor for a month or so which showed cardiac arrhythmia; now I have a pacemaker.

'It's probably the drugs,' Des told me when we discussed the cardiologist's findings. 'The suite of medicines you've been prescribed is known to disturb the heart rhythm in some patients.'

It's not absolutely clear that it was my heart that caused the blackout, but it seemed expedient to keep off the roads from now on. This issue has never been resolved, so my driving days are well and truly over.

As the year continued to play itself out, I was focusing on finding a gentler frame of mind, but suffered occasional dips into frustration. This was, I believe, unavoidable, as my functioning was slowly yet steadily deteriorating.

Miriam has shared in my descent from clarity every step of the way. Always in my corner, watching out for me, she observes and monitors the progression of the disease with extreme care. I see this; I see it registering in her eyes, but she rarely comments. Being sensitive, she springs into action in order to spare my blushes, and I'm grateful to her. I suspect that Miriam knows the score far better than I do. She observes, I struggle, and can no longer see the full picture because I can't remember what that picture is.

And of course, life at home is not all harmony. We have clashes, and heated exchanges about domestic planning and tasks; but the underlying stress is worry for the future. How can you live well in the present when the future appears so challenging for Miriam, and for me? We have individual moments of being on edge, stressed and fretful.

Whenever life seems particularly difficult we take ourselves off for a weekend of pampering. This time we were away in Lough Rynn Castle in Leitrim, a treat that had been a gift from Hannah. As we sat in front of the fire enjoying our pre-dinner drinks, I told Miriam how low I was feeling about the Alzheimer's. 'It's just relentlessly progressing,' I said. 'Like a runaway lorry with no brakes.'

Squeezing my hand she said that she understood how I felt. 'But we're here now,' she said. 'And now is restful. It's relaxing. Nurturing. Let's just take that for now. Deal?'

I smiled and, lifting my glass to hers, agreed, 'Deal!'

And I did manage to relax into it all, knowing that once we got home again it would be back to fighting the good fight. Back to grieving.

Grief was a *big* factor: grief for the future we had believed was ours; for the present; and the things we have already lost. Miriam tries for my sake to keep her sadness private, but on the rare times when it spills over and she weeps in my presence, I welcome her honesty. She shares my worst moments too.

This is an intimately shared journey – carer and patient yoked firmly together. We look out for each other, trying to do our very best.

One inevitable, and decidedly unwelcome, change was that Miriam and I had swapped roles. She was learning to take over various tasks in order that I could avoid unnecessary stress. And so it was that, when we took a bargain-basement weekend break in Berlin – a city that was new to us both – Miriam took charge of all the logistics.

She made the travel arrangements, booked the accommodation and selected what we should see, where we should go and how we would get there. Neither of us mentioned this transfer of power out loud, but we were both aware that this was good practice for our new and future reality.

It was a great trip, but there were stressful moments as Miriam grappled with her new role. When this happened, when she struggled to navigate the public transport system or lost her way, I tried hard to be helpful. But I suspect my fumbling, last-minute interventions were more of a hindrance than a help. Nevertheless we returned home, happy in the knowledge that the first step on the experimentation to discover a solid path through the change in our roles had been achieved.

There is no doubt that my advocacy with the Alzheimer Society of Ireland (ASI) was still advantageous to me, as well as to others, if only to gain hope for the improvements research might bring. The situation, I had learned, wasn't entirely bleak. Science is hard at work and making some headway. There is a new field in gene therapy, for example, in which there is direct intervention in re-engineering genes. Clustered Regularly Interspaced Short Palindromic Repeats (CRISPR), a method of treating the condition, is looking increasingly more achievable and effective.

But there were times when, listening to the best experts, I was hit over the head with a loss of hope.

At one conference, for example, the expert scientific researcher into the pathology of Alzheimer's was making it abundantly clear that if there was a breakthrough treatment, it was highly improbable that it could reverse the damage that had already been done. It would only stop further decline.

Thinking of all the work I had put into slowing the incremental process, of all the exercise, the diet and the cognitive challenges I'd set myself in order to stave off the worst, I felt winded. I'd done all that and still the illness had progressed. Damage had accumulated. A successful treatment, therefore, could merely keep me frozen in a debilitated state for a longer time. What fun was that? What value?

These dark thoughts were tumbling through my mind when I heard the Chair mention my name. 'Now Ronan Smith will give his talk of positivity and hope,' he said, and my heart sank.

Feeling like a charlatan, I rattled through my routine trying to sound sincere, while my head spun with the ugly reality. I was talking of my hope to raise the bar, and hope for a cure that is not just a halt in decline, when the expert's words had drained my hope away in a heartbeat. It now seemed a naïve and unlikely notion.

Returning home with a heavy heart, I decided I would prefer a steady decline and no such plateau. 'That,' I thought, 'would be better both for myself and for my family.'

In June, Loughlin and I flew to Spain to walk the final stage of the Camino route, ending up in Santiago de Compostela. This had been Miriam's idea, a chance for me and Loughlin to spend time together and bond. I was very aware of being minded; Loughlin was the route finder, the man in charge, walking a few steps ahead of me, but I followed like a happy sheep, aware that I needed Loughlin's able traveller instincts.

As we walked each day, we talked. We talked of faith, and he told me he is an atheist. This certainty surprised me. We talked of the future, what the illness was likely to bring

213

to me and what was in store for him in years to come. There was a time when I wondered if Loughlin would follow me into theatre work. He has natural acting and comedic talent, but it's not where his passion lies. It was always art for him. From the time when he was aged eleven, and Miriam took him into the National College of Art and Design (NCAD) and a friend of hers, a tutor there, showed him round, he had considered no other profession.

He has changed his course at NCAD several times, and is unsure of which direction in art he should take. Talking of my own career, and of how abandoning law in favour of acting had worked out well for me, I reassured him. 'Just follow your passion,' I said, 'and it will all become clear. It'll work out. You'll see.'

Miriam was right. It was wonderful spending time with my son, a real bonding experience. He is an easy, engaging companion, and we chatted happily to each other and to all the travellers we met along the way as we walked. They were charmed by him, this hidden atheist who was accompanied by a demented and challenged father!

In late summer I was flying off again. Miriam and I were given a wonderful opportunity. We were asked to attend a conference in Tuscany along with Cathy, a fellow member of the working team of the ASI. It was an initiative carried out by the Italian government in association with Ulster University, Coleraine. People were to attend from all over the world: scientists and academics, and the 'guinea pigs,' of which I was one – as was Miriam, although, she, of course, was there to represent carers.

By engaging with us, these people would be better placed to work in the field of dementia. As members of the team, the ASI had tasked us with finding out how other countries managed Alzheimer's. When we reached Pisa Airport Cathy said, 'We should ask for assistance.'

Miriam was surprised. 'I know we had it in Dublin,' she said, 'but surely we don't need it here, this is a tiny airport.' But Cathy explained that it was an exercise. And that she and I had to check out the systems at various airports. Dublin had passed with flying colours, but we wanted to find out what policies Italy had in place for airline travellers with the disease.

Cathy went up to these two airport officials standing on the tarmac outside having a fag, and she said, '*Buongiorno*, we need assistance.'

They looked her up and down and then glanced over at Miriam and me. And presumably thinking that we all looked terribly well and were walking smartly, they looked confused but gamely said, '*Sì, sì, sì*. And what is the disability?'

'Dementia.'

Nodding, and without hesitation, one of them, a woman, marched up to Miriam, took her arm and led her through the airport. Cathy and I looked at each other and, laughing, followed on behind.

When we got to the baggage area the woman stood a few feet away. Miriam turned to Cathy and said, 'I bet you fifty bucks when we've got our bags she'll take my arm again.'

Miriam won her bet. She was marched out of the door with us behind, bent over with laughter.

When we caught up with Miriam the woman was saying in pidgin English, 'You are on holidays?'

Anxious to keep the exchange simple Miriam said, '*Sì*.'

'And where are you going?'

Miriam answered, 'I have no idea.' And before she had time to explain that we were off for a workshop and she didn't know quite where it was based the woman, looking embarrassed said, 'Oh, I understand.'

We looked at each other, feeling sorry for that poor woman who obviously believed that, in asking someone with dementia where they were going, she had been irredeemably insensitive. But soon laughter overcame us again, and we were still chuckling when our friends Eloisa and Christian arrived and collected us.

We had a wonderful week! We stayed in a Medici castle and had wonderful food and great craic. It felt like a holiday. It *was* essentially a holiday. Except that we felt useful. Sadness and fear did not exist that week. They gave way to fun and laughter.

I've become cranky. I don't like that. It's a characteristic I dislike in others and can't bear to see in myself. It takes me by surprise, making me feel like a stranger to myself. I walk now with two dogs. I presented Bella, a Cockapoo, to Miriam on her last birthday. She is a fluffy ball of energy and a pure delight.

Pepsi puts up with her. But he's old now, and is losing his memory too. On our walks he lifts a leg to urinate, then drops it, then raises the other one before doing a three-hundred-and-sixty-degree turn. I truly empathise with him.

I'm still working with the ASI. It continues to give me a sense of purpose. And through my work there, along with my own journey, I'm learning to better understand my father. His Alzheimer's story, and my ongoing one, are chalk and cheese. Perhaps each story is to some degree a creature of its times, but my father had chosen an impossible path – one that actually did not exist.

He put himself through a punishing, fretful, stressful struggle, and ended up being something of an empty vessel. But in being empty he was, at least, calm. He smiled at the end. That has always been a comfort to me.

My story to date is quite different. By engaging with Alzheimer's, by learning all I could, I am in a much better place to deal with each difficulty as it arises. What is my future? I can't know that. But I have to hang on to optimism. And at the end of the year, on a plane coming back from a conference in Barcelona, I found a reason to be hopeful.

Miriam and I were sitting together, with a young woman in the window seat. While Miriam and I read, this woman was focused on her computer, tapping rapidly and intensely. Then towards the end of the flight, she closed her computer and put it away. Her elbow bumped my arm.

'I'm sorry,' she said.

'That's quite all right.' Smiling at her, pointing at her laptop I said, 'I'm impressed with your diligent industry.'

The three of us started a conversation, and she told us that she was a research scientist in the medical field.

'That's interesting,' I said. 'What area of medicine is that?'

'I work in gene therapy.'

My ears pricked. I told her about my diagnosis, explaining that I had the genetic form of Alzheimer's. 'What's the current thinking in the global community about the prospect of a cure?'

Turning, she looked me in the eye and said, 'There will be a cure for Alzheimer's within ten years.'

'You sound very certain,' I said.

'All my international colleagues believe it,' she said. 'The momentum is regarded as unstoppable.'

At that moment the captain announced that we would be landing shortly, and should put on our safety belts and return our seats to the upright position.

Aware that my time to quiz her was short I blurted out, 'Where might that leave me?'

She looked at me questioningly.

'I mean, surely that cure will be too late for me? My cognitive ability is already compromised, and the damage is mounting at a quickening pace.'

'Ah,' she said, 'but in parallel with finding a preventative cure, we will also be able to restore function to damaged brains.'

'Really?' I was holding my breath.

'Yes. We hope to generate new, healthy brain cells containing the patient's exact profile.'

'And you'll implant those?' asked Miriam, leaning across my seat.

She nodded. 'Exactly!'

As we flew over Howth and began our descent with the lovely image of Dublin Bay to our left, my heart felt lighter than it had in years. The Beast may yet be defeated.

Throughout this dementia journey I have been writing this book. Conceived primarily to spread awareness, it has proved useful as a cognitive challenge. It's been an enjoyable enterprise and has complemented my advocacy work with the ASI.

However, the truth is that as time passes the writing has become harder. It gets slower in a mechanical sense, and

I'm struggling with my spelling. Try as I might – and I do try – to tough it out, and retrieve the spelled word from my memory (I can't let the Beast win the battle every time), I have to check my words more and more frequently. And, where once writing came naturally to me, now I scan the thesaurus, fussing and fretting as I find the best possible word to use.

Enough! Now that the pleasure of it has turned sour on me, I've decided to stop. I'm happy with that. These days, as another year draws to a close, I become stressed at the drop of a hat; it takes less and less to send my mood into a downward spiral. By making more space for myself and letting go of commitments, I can better contain that stress.

And although this tale of two dementia stories isn't quite over, not yet, my telling of it is.

Nineteen

A Day in Miriam's Life: November 2020

If I had one wish, I would go back to a day in 1991. It was winter, and Ronan and I were in India on a belated honeymoon. Bangaram Island is one of the tiniest, most beautiful islands in an archipelago in the Indian Ocean. It has white sands, azure sea and a three-kilometre warm lagoon surrounding it, and it became the christening place of my first ever swim.

As a non-swimmer I had a fear of water, but that lagoon, with its exotic collection of sea life of all the colours of the rainbow, became my safe place. We navigated the water, threading the seabed while boxfish, clownfish, and yellow tang caressed our ankles.

Ronan held me each day, his hand under my tummy, giving me confidence. Our last day on the island, feeling as though I was ready to try to swim alone, I asked him to let go. And I swam! I couldn't believe it. I was swimming in the Indian Ocean! I was ecstatic. I could see Ronan's legs keeping pace beside me, guiding me gently, as he has continued to do through our thirty years of marriage.

It's so good to remember that time now, on this November day twenty-nine years later when, in Covid-19 lockdown, we navigate a very different ocean. I am guiding Ronan while we live with this Beast, and every time I look at him, I see another bit gone.

I am his carer. But how I *hate* that word. To me, a carer is a person generally employed by the state to give a half to one hour a day of personal care. It's someone who comes in, wipes your bum, showers you and leaves.

In 2018, when I arrived in accident and emergency after Ronan's car crash, the nurse, looking at me said, 'Are you his carer?'

'Yes, I'm his carer,' I said. 'But I'm also his wife, and his best friend. His right hand, his decision-maker, parent to his lovely children.'

She smiled, a little embarrassed.

'Yes,' I said with resignation. 'I'm his carer.'

Living with Ronan today is very different from living with him a month ago, and *that* was very different from living with him six months ago.

I wake at around seven o'clock to find our younger dog, Bella, scratching on the door to be let out. After letting her into the garden, I make tea and go back to bed. Ronan is still asleep. Then I get up and make breakfast for both of us. A year ago Ronan made his own breakfast; eighteen months ago he made an excellent omelette, but that has changed. I place the honey and peanut butter in an obvious place, where Ronan will see the jars. Last week he could find them himself, but not now, and I don't want to disempower him. I have to think ahead all the time.

He comes into the kitchen dressed, but wearing two shirts. I place his clothes out for him each night, but he gets mixed up even with that. He gets distracted. I put out nice clothes but sometimes he puts on his working clothes and that is silly, he never works in the garden now.

After breakfast Ronan takes Bella for a walk. I suggest it and put the lead in his hand. This is new. Ronan's speech has deteriorated; he finds it hard to form a sentence. When he wants to say, 'I think I'll take Bella out because it's going to rain later,' he'll say, 'I think . . . rain.' The thought starts the sentence, but the syntax has gone. It's dreadful for him.

It takes him a while to get ready to go out, but he loves his walks, and takes two most days. He has three routes. I don't worry that he'll get lost. Not at the moment. He always comes back safely.

Today, the moment he arrives back and comes into the kitchen he switches the kettle on. That's instinctive. A few weeks ago he would have made the tea, but today, I make it. We sit down and drink it at the kitchen table. If it was fine, we'd go out onto the deck to watch the clouds and the birds. Nature is a big thing in Ronan's life, and in mine.

Tea finished, Ronan doesn't know what to do with himself. He no longer has the ability to say, 'I'm bored, I must do something.' His brain no longer works like that. I owe it to him to be his brain.

I might say, 'Go and sit by the fire and read the *National Geographic*.' Or I did until recently, but now his cognition has worsened. Now I hold his hand, bring him to the couch and put the *National Geographic* in his hand.

Preparing the lunch, I ponder on my growing awareness that expectation and disappointment are intrinsically linked. A few years ago, when Ronan's memory was beginning to fail, I used to get frustrated; and, worse than that, annoyed, angry and confused. I couldn't come to terms with the fact that Ronan was either refusing or, if he attempted them, failing to do certain tasks. It's one of the cruellest aspects of Alzheimer's. No amount of research, reading or talking to medics prepares you for the fact that each day brings subtle changes.

I've now learned that, in order to cope, I have to let go of any expectation of Ronan. When I do that there is no anger, no confusion and, above all, no disappointment. No expectation equals no disappointment.

It was, for example, Ronan's job to set the table. If I ask him to set it I'll have to ask him ten times, and these days, he can't do it. If I persisted in asking, it would cause me stress, grief, anger and disappointment, but if I set it myself that helps my sanity.

I am so aware of that now. I have to catch myself every time I feel like saying, 'But you *know* how to do that!' Just because Ronan could do something yesterday doesn't necessarily mean he can do it today. Because of that I try to live my day consciously, almost like morning meditation. I'll think, 'How is today going to be?' I'll make sure it's not too full of my expectation, and I try to pre-empt any difficulty. It's not an easy task, but it's a useful tool for building a loving, accepting home for all of us involved.

I'm Ronan's dietitian now and we eat well. Our diet contains a lot of fish, and vegetables and fruit from the garden. The freezer is full of beans and raspberries. For lunch I make an omelette with salad. Ronan is a fantastic eater, and he's very appreciative of everything I give him. He's very grateful. Imagine if he wasn't?

After lunch, at around 2 p.m., Ronan will go for a rest. Now I go and lie down with him. I say, 'Handies', and he says, 'Handies', and we just lie there, holding hands. That's a hard time. Because as we lie there, gazing into each other's eyes, it's as if we are saying a silent goodbye. When a friend asked me recently what the hardest thing was for me, that was the example I gave. That, and witnessing his sadness and confusion; his awareness of his condition. Ronan drifts into sleep and I stay in the moment, being mindful; no longer looking into the future, because that spells devastation.

I get up first and go to the kitchen to make tea and toast. I take it in to Ronan. He gives me a cheeky grin and says, 'When does your shift finish?' I love that. It's a chink of the old Ronan – back to being playful with me. In the past we were always slagging each other.

We need more wood for the fire. I can't carry it because I have a bad back, but I can no longer say, 'Ronan darling, would you take the basket, go outside and bring in some wood?' Not now. I have to keep my sentences short and to the point. I take the empty basket out to the log pile and say, 'Fill that. Good man.' But I can't say, 'Fill that and bring it back to me,' because that gets him agitated. I now wait until the basket is full and then ask him to carry it in. That's a new development, it's happened in the past two weeks.

The children say, 'You've got to give yourself a rest Mummy. You can't be watching his every mood and taking responsibility for his confusion,' but I do, because I love him so much.

When I see panic and sadness in his eyes that makes me really upset. But there are times he is happy, and when he is, I'm happy too. I bought him a ping-pong set during early lockdown to use on the kitchen table. Our lovely neighbours, Bryan and Caroline, visit frequently for a bash around – they're in our lockdown bubble.

Ronan is immediately transported back in time. To a time when he was fun-loving, dramatic and agile. Ronan was a superb fencer. As a student he represented Ireland twice, along with his friend Philip Lee. That sharpness and deep focus needed for the sport he can, astonishingly, access now, when playing ping-pong. He's alert, happy and highly competitive.

It helps, I think, that ping-pong is an activity that doesn't require dialogue. He can partake equally with others. It's an utter transformation. He's dramatic, shouting and laughing. It's his happy drug, and he is transformed into the old Ronan.

There are other times I see that spark. He'll come out with a John B. Keane accent and phrase to make me, and others, laugh. He can still perform! It's second nature to him.

At six o'clock I turn on the TV and Ronan watches the news. I give him his dinner, and I eat mine, alone in the kitchen. That's part of the loneliness of being a carer. I could eat with Ronan, but it's lonely eating with someone who doesn't speak to you. That is stressful and makes me want to cry. You're looking at the person who you love, but who has left you.

Television distracts Ronan. He can't switch it on himself anymore, and after dinner I put on *Dad's Army* on a loop. He could watch that forever! It's tapping into his memories. He watched it as a child when, in his mind, his father was the blustering Captain Mainwaring. It's another happiness drug.

Ronan used to love *Cracker*, or a thriller heist, but he can't follow that now. He loves *Father Ted*, and his face comes alive when he's watching a programme about chimpanzees. He smiles and laughs out loud. He loves all animals, but especially chimps, because they are so childlike and playful.

While he's watching I'll be next door, washing up. I'll give Ronan his meds, then I might listen to *Arena*, the arts show on RTÉ Radio, and do some felting, or make a few phone calls to friends. That contact keeps me sane. I have choir every Tuesday on Zoom – that's another lifeline. I could not be without my good friends, and I'm blessed with our neighbours.

The children are amazing. They're both settled and happy now. Hannah is a primary school teacher, a job she adores, and Loughlin has found great success as a sign painter and graphic designer since leaving NCAD. He talks of it with excitement on his weekend visits.

'It's so varied,' he says. 'Last week I was in Tipperary painting a name onto someone's yacht, and this week I painted a huge mural in the offices of a video game company.'

Hannah lives in Ashford, Co. Wicklow, and Loughlin in Dublin. Both children visit us every weekend which is wonderful for me, but can be particularly tough for them. Seeing their father with a gap of a week means that they see the deterioration most starkly. When Hannah's boyfriend James visited with her recently, he said to her afterwards, 'Your dad was in great form.' She had to explain to him that in company, over dinner, Ronan can still put on a performance.

He hadn't been there when Hannah asked Ronan to put the milk in the fridge. 'Mum, he couldn't do it,' she said to me, clearly distressed. 'He stared at the milk for a while. Then he picked it up, and took it through to the sitting room.'

The next time she came he was trying to eat his soup with a fork. Although losing her daddy is the worst thing for Hannah, she is endlessly patient with him. 'I love him so much,' she said when I commented on this. 'And it breaks my heart that he is not happy in himself. I hate that he is aware that his cognition is failing. I hate seeing his frustration.'

Loughlin has inherited Ronan's ability to act out a story. He can be funny, and I know he finds it hard now that his father has lost this ability. 'There's so much sadness in that,' he says. 'And I hate having to tell him what to do. Giving him an order sounds so harsh, but suggestion doesn't seem to work.'

Ronan's friends have been wonderful: Philip Lee, Julian Erskine and other colleagues from his theatre days. Everyone says the same thing – that Ronan was wonderful at his job; that with his clear-cut legal mind he always saw the real problem, and dealt with that; that he managed clashing egos with ease; that he was a brilliant negotiator who was always, unfailingly, extraordinarily fair. He was also great fun. The best ever company.

Julian Erskine says he'll be remembered for never taking sides in his dealings with people, and never showing favour. 'He was the perfect person to come into *Riverdance* and put a sense of order and fairness into the leaping contractual elements. But I'll remember him best as a family man,' he said. 'He was sensitive. In an office where the show was the thing, and the show must go on, Ronan always had a picture of Hannah and Loughlin on his desk. I remember thinking, there is a man with his priorities in the right order.

'Hannah and Loughlin are gorgeous people,' he said, 'and they're a product of you and Ronan. And of everything

Ronan did for them. His sacrifice was to give them the right education, to make sure that they could be what they wanted to be, freed from any shackle.' Hearing that made us both so happy.

Ronan goes to bed around nine-thirty or ten o'clock. Sometimes, if I'm tired or in pain with my arthritis, I'll go earlier. One evening, lying there all cosy, I was dying of thirst. When Ronan appeared I said, 'Sweetheart, will you get me a glass of water?'

He looked at me and said, very slowly, 'A glass. Of water.' It's by repeating things simply and slowly that he remembers them. Or tries to.

Ten minutes later the door opened. It was Ronan – but no water. I repeated my request and, nodding, he said again, 'A glass. Of water.'

I heard him walking up and down and asked him a third time. And then I heard the tap running. That, I felt, was a good sign. But then he walked straight past the bedroom door and continued down the corridor! 'Sweetheart,' I said, 'I'm up here.'

'Up here?' He sounded confused. 'Up where?'

'I'm here, sweetheart, in the bed.'

'I. Am. Coming.' He came right up to the bedroom door, holding the glass of water, and looked in. 'What's the matter, Miriam?' he asked.

'I just want a glass of water.'

'Yes, I know,' he said. 'And I am looking for you.' And, on a mission, he walked away from me down the corridor.

I laughed so much then, because you have to enjoy the funny side of Alzheimer's if you want to stay sane. And when I re-enacted the scene for Ronan, who had no memory of it, he was in stitches too! There is so much humour in Alzheimer's, and you have to get your laughs wherever you can.

Another evening the phone rang and, hearing that it was someone whose conversation drains my energy, I told Ronan to say that I was asleep in bed. Confused by the video call, Ronan pointed the screen towards me, showing the caller that I was sitting there in the chair. 'Miriam can't come to the phone,' he said. 'She says she's asleep in bed.'

A farce of epic proportions ensued as, dropping to the floor, I crept around trying to stay out of sight, as Ronan followed my every step. Wanting to watch TV I tried to push Ronan, still on the phone, into the kitchen. He kicked out at me. Then I rang the doorbell, telling Ronan he now had an excuse to end the call. But he went outside and announced, loudly, that there was nobody there. And then, to confuse matters still further, he said to the caller, 'Miriam says that your doorbell is ringing. You need to get off the phone.' You really couldn't make it up!

I had a friend whose husband died from Alzheimer's. He was on holiday with her once, and she took him to the toilet in the restaurant. Fifteen minutes later he hadn't returned to the table, and my friend opened the toilet door, to see him just standing there. She asked him what he was doing.

'It's hard to pee when there's a man staring at you,' he said, gazing steadily into a mirror. 'Mind you,' he added, 'he *is* rather handsome!'

But it's not all laughs. When I'm lying in bed beside Ronan I am screaming inside. Absolutely screaming, 'Don't leave me!' It's more grief than rage – I feel terrified, and sad. And sometimes we cry together, the noise dreadful – like a cow in distress – roaring crying together. There's nothing to say, but we're on the same page.

Sometimes I imagine what it would be like to be married to someone with Alzheimer's who you really did not like. You would have all of the frustration, and all the one-way street, with you giving to him, and nothing coming back. Imagine! I know people in really crappy marriages, and that is sad. I'm in a dark world of constant worry, pain and grief, but I really love Ronan, and Ronan loves me. I think of myself as his lover and wife, but someone who also cares for him. He is my very best friend. I cannot imagine how I am going to be in the world without him.

Acknowledgements

It takes a large team to produce a book. I would like to thank all my family and friends, and the professionals who have helped to bring my memoir into being.

Thanks to my brother, Julian Smith, the family's only non-thespian, who has assisted me with all the dreaded new technology. To Philip Lee, my lifelong friend, who has given such practical, emotional and legal support. To the eminent geriatrician, Professor Des O'Neill, for passing on invaluable expert medical advice, friendship and practical help in the years since my diagnosis. To Ian Robertson, professor emeritus at Trinity College Dublin, for his counsel and friendship. To my neighbour Bryan Sullivan, who has always been there when we needed him. To Martin Drury, my friend and colleague whose support has never wavered, and to Julian Erskine whose friendship means so much, and who, in practical ways, has brought fun into our lives.

I'd like to thank my agent Sallyanne Sweeney, writer Sue Leonard, and all at New Island Books, especially Aoife K. Walsh, Susan McKeever and Caoimhe Fox.

But most of all I thank my wonderful wife and soulmate, Miriam Brady, who has travelled with me every step of the way, and our beautiful, talented children, Hannah and Loughlin, who are my greatest legacy.

Index